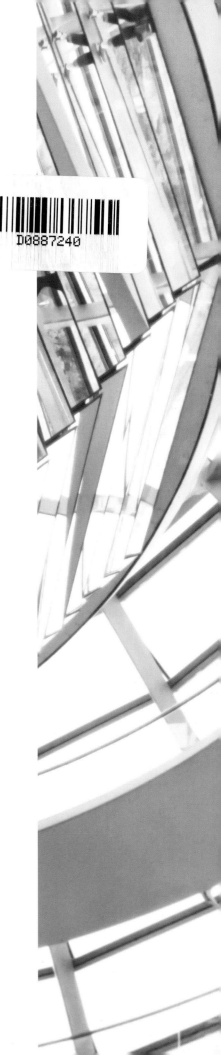

FUTURESCAN™
Healthcare Trends and Implications
2016–2021

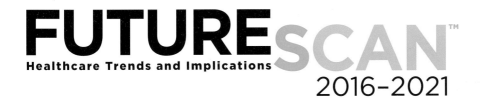

CONTENTS

A Guide to Using *Futurescan*

by Don Seymour

The goal of *Futurescan* is to assist leaders in more accurately forecasting whether current and emerging trends will "stick" and have an important impact on their healthcare organization (Gladwell 2000). Every year, eight industry thought leaders are invited to look to the future and share their insights and predictions. Based on the results of the latest *Futurescan* survey, each article presents the author's assumptions regarding the "stickiness" of a particular trend, as well as specific implications for providers.

With the help of *Futurescan*, executives can use the following methodology as part of their planning process to analyze factors that might influence their organization and develop strategies to address them:

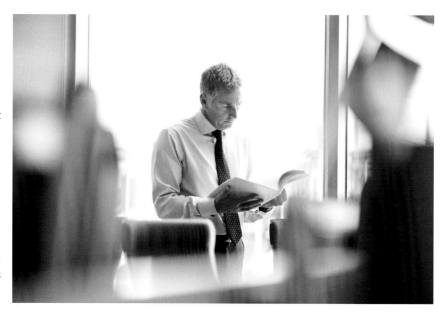

1. Separate external trends that often cannot be controlled from internal trends and operational issues that frequently can be controlled.
2. Build consensus among senior leaders regarding the most important trends and their stickiness.
3. Reach agreement on the potential opportunities and threats the trends present.
4. Determine appropriate action steps to capitalize on the opportunities and minimize the threats.
5. Establish a system for measuring the results and monitoring the trends.

Futurescan is intended to be a valuable resource for implementing this approach and positioning organizations for success in the ever-changing healthcare landscape.

Reference

Gladwell, M. 2000. *The Tipping Point: How Little Things Can Make a Big Difference.* New York: Little, Brown and Company.

About the Author

Don Seymour, president of Don Seymour & Associates in Winchester, Massachusetts, has been a strategy adviser to health system boards, senior executives, and medical staff leaders for 30 years. A frequent presenter on subjects related to senior leadership in healthcare organizations, he has served on the faculties of the American College of Healthcare Executives and The Governance Institute. Additionally, he has made presentations to the American Hospital Association; Fortune 100 companies; and a variety of other national, state, and regional groups. He previously served as executive editor of *Futurescan*. A past president of the Society for Healthcare Strategy & Market Development, he received its Award for Individual Professional Excellence in 2008.

Got Change? Transformation in the Healthcare Marketplace

by Ian Morrison, PhD

Got change? *Futurescan 2016–2021* focuses on the key dimensions of change in the rapidly transforming healthcare marketplace. All strategy professionals need to deepen their understanding of these critical developments and incorporate key learnings into their ongoing work in innovation, strategic planning, marketing, and communications.

From my perspective, the US healthcare system is now in "high change mode." We have done the PowerPoint version. Now we are making it real and facing the future—even if keeping up is a struggle. Fortunately, the outstanding guest contributors to this year's report have provided some key insights that will help us navigate the new environment.

Volume to Value

The transition from volume to value is being fueled by new payment models that reached a tipping point in 2015 as both public and private purchasers pressed forward with increased emphasis on value-based payment and accountable care. All of the contributors underscore the importance of this trend in the themes they have analyzed for *Futurescan*:

- The need to engage increasingly value-conscious consumers

- The strategic capital model required to finance the evolving healthcare system
- The change leadership competencies necessary for the future
- The imperative to accelerate innovation that improves value
- The need to implement transformations at a massive scale, such as in the Veterans Administration
- The renewed focus on health promotion and wellness programs that work
- The migration to risk for defined populations
- The call to integrate behavioral health and medical care

Our distinguished contributors shed light on how healthcare executives view these issues through the lens of the *Futurescan* survey. They also discuss how strategists should respond. Here are some key highlights.

The patient experience: Healthcare increasingly resembles a retail industry, with consumers picking insurance plans and shopping for medical services. In light of this trend, Christy Dempsey of Press Ganey encourages providers to take a broad view of the patient experience that encompasses "the clinical, operational, cultural, and behavioral aspects of services provided across the continuum of care." Because HCAHPS

(Hospital Consumer Assessment of Healthcare Providers and Systems) ratings are tied to reimbursement and now account for 30 percent of a hospital's value-based purchasing score, it is more important than ever for health systems to measure, manage, and improve the patient experience. Accomplishing this goal, according to Dempsey, will require doctors, nurses, and other employees to be actively engaged in a team-based approach to care.

Capital fuel for transformation: Major capital will be needed to underwrite the cost of the massive changes in healthcare, and both not-for-profit and for-profit financial markets will play a role. To execute an effective business model migration, providers will need to get the math right on strategic capital. Michael Irwin of Citi explains the new healthcare capital environment in terms of broader developments in the industry, such as the growth of ambulatory care and physician networks, the need to fund an information technology infrastructure, the rise of joint ventures, and the assumption of risk by providers.

Irwin suggests that traditional tax-exempt bond financing may be in conflict with emerging trends. This conflict may require health systems to consider nontraditional funding sources, including taxable corporate debt and taxable private placements. As these trends play

About the Author

Ian Morrison, PhD, is an author, a consultant, and a futurist. He received an undergraduate degree from the University of Edinburgh, Scotland; a graduate degree from the University of Newcastle upon Tyne, England; and an interdisciplinary doctorate in urban studies from the University of British Columbia, Canada. He is the author of several books, including the best-selling *The Second Curve: Managing the Velocity of Change*. Morrison is the former president of the Institute for the Future and a founding partner of Strategic Health Perspectives, a forecasting service for clients in the healthcare industry.

out, Irwin anticipates that operating effectiveness and scale will be critical factors in securing the financing needed to fuel healthcare's transformation.

Leading change: As the incentives shift, as organizations merge, and as new entrants threaten old ways of doing things, executives need to adapt to the evolving healthcare landscape. Change expert Todd D. Jick, PhD, of Columbia Business School reminds us that all industries are going through significant transitions and that the "winners will be the executives who can best manage and lead their organization through a world of continuous change." Jick emphasizes three critical components of change leadership:

1. Managing new business models
2. Managing organizational forms, consolidations, and partnerships
3. Upgrading leadership competencies

The good news is that change leadership can be learned and that those who embrace the new skills are more likely to succeed.

Harnessing and accelerating innovation: Transformation for higher performance is tough to achieve in any industry. In healthcare it is doubly difficult because of relentless advances in medical science and the demands of an aging, sicker society. A key to solving this conundrum is harnessing innovations that can improve quality and reduce costs and bringing them to scale by accelerating the adoption of promising technologies.

Ezra Mehlman of Health Enterprise Partners points out that "health systems have begun to find new growth opportunities by experimenting with investment and innovation programs, or accelerators." Mehlman highlights four goals driving the creation of these programs:

1. Achieving financial returns by taking equity stakes in growth-minded companies
2. Improving core healthcare operations

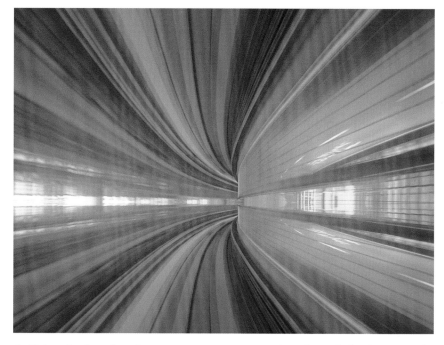

3. Enhancing brand equity
4. Cultivating an innovation-focused culture

The *Futurescan* survey results provide evidence of the trend toward innovation, which Mehlman says offers several key insights:

- A new paradigm has emerged of health systems working with early-stage companies.
- An internal resource commitment is essential.
- The right structure for an innovation program depends on an organization's objectives and risk appetite.
- Revenue diversification is the name of the game.

Transforming at scale: Transformation cannot occur just at the edges. It has to be deep, wide reaching, and massive in scale. Lessons can be learned from giants on that journey, such as the US Department of Veterans Affairs (VA). VA Secretary Robert A. McDonald emphasizes the power of

- partnerships, in the VA's fight against homelessness among veterans;
- preparation, in anticipating massive increases in the number of veterans with dementia;

- prevention, through the department's focus on health and wellness; and
- prediction, in forecasting the needs of the future VA population through analytics and genetics.

Promoting health: Proactive efforts to promote health and wellness will increasingly move the healthcare paradigm away from sick care. Making this shift a reality will involve effort and investment from all stakeholders, especially patients. Michael F. Roizen, MD, and Olivia Delia of Cleveland Clinic emphasize that "more than 80 percent of the nation's $2.5 trillion health spend goes to chronic disease management." These diseases include "lifestyle-induced conditions that take the lives of more than seven in ten Americans, such as type 2 diabetes, dementia, cancer, osteoarthritis, heart disease, and stroke."

Roizen and Delia highlight Cleveland Clinic's efforts to motivate people to achieve normal ranges for low density lipoprotein cholesterol, blood pressure, blood sugar, waist-to-height ratio, stress management, and tobacco toxins. Research shows that achieving these "six normals," with or without medication, reduces subsequent chronic disease by 80 to 90 percent over 10- to 30-year periods.

The Cleveland Clinic model emphasizes

- transforming an organization's culture under the leadership of the CEO,
- changing the environment to support health (e.g., creating tobacco-free campuses, influencing eating choices),
- establishing coordinated-care programs,
- creating social and fun activities to encourage health, and
- fueling it all with meaningful financial incentives.

This model has allowed Cleveland Clinic to dramatically improve the health of its own employees and dependents while reducing costs. As the authors conclude, "If only 65 percent of individuals achieved the six normals, the nation would save well over $600 billion in healthcare spending per year." Currently, only 3 to 4 percent of the US population entering Medicare is there.

Migration to risk: As a result of the volume-to-value shift, many health systems are on a journey to bear more risk for the cost and quality of care. Managing this risk changes the incentives, the objectives, the capital needs, and the skills now required of providers. The combined growth of Medicare Advantage plans, accountable care organizations, bundled payments, and consumerism will challenge all health systems to focus on value. Lee B. Sacks, MD, and Michael J. Randall, FACHE, of Advocate Health Care review these drivers and point out some effective ways to address them, including identifying the best paths to risk assumption. They encourage leaders to "recognize they are better off shaping their own future than waiting for it to happen."

Behavioral health: As the industry migrates to population health and risk management, leaders are realizing that behavioral health is often at the heart of complex and expensive medical issues. Further, now that mental health parity has been achieved through legislation, it is vital for health systems to integrate behavioral health into their core offerings.

M. Justin Coffey, MD, and C. Edward Coffey, MD, of Menninger Clinic note that "one in five Americans suffers from one or more mental disorders" and emphasize that comorbidity of mental disorders and general medical disorders is the rule rather than the exception. They are heartened that *Futurescan* respondents see an increased focus on this issue, noting that "models of integrated care exist . . . and have been shown to work for adults as well as for children and adolescents." Drs. Coffey and Coffey also highlight the importance of effective information management in behavioral healthcare. They advocate

- establishment of a fully transparent medical record,
- design of medical records that facilitate the collection of behavioral and psychosocial information, and
- creation of a pragmatic approach to screening for mental health conditions.

Conclusion

A new era in healthcare is here. Strategists must help health systems navigate the change waters to create high-performing organizations that meet the needs of patients, payers, and providers. The voyage will require a deep understanding of the emerging trends, a focused analysis of what matters most, and an ability to translate industry intelligence into actionable strategies. Change can be overwhelming, but in my travels I see leaders stepping up to the challenge. They are increasingly energized to overcome obstacles and seek out new opportunities to serve their communities in the evolving healthcare environment.

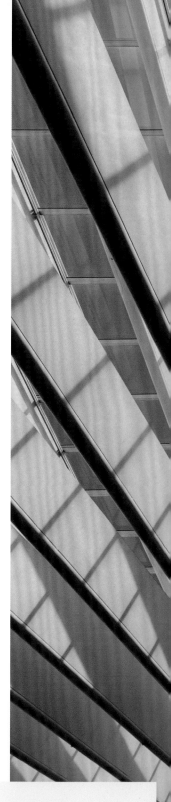

The Evolution of the Patient Experience

by Christy Dempsey

Healthcare executives have long been focused on patient satisfaction scores. The primary reason for soliciting feedback from patients has always been a desire to improve hospitals and healthcare systems by better understanding and meeting the needs of patients and their families. Today, administrators, physicians, nurses, and other healthcare providers are shifting their attention from the "soft" aspects of patient satisfaction to the totality of the patient experience, which encompasses the clinical, operational, cultural, and behavioral aspects of services provided across the continuum of care.

Patient Satisfaction Versus Patient Experience

Historically, the term "patient satisfaction" connoted a superficial metric that could be improved with a mere smile as a staff member closed curtains for privacy or delivered the daily newspaper to patients during their hospital stay. Now when we speak of measuring the "patient experience," we take into account the totality of the experience of all people who enter our facilities, whether they are healthy or sick.

The patient experience incorporates *every* facet of care provided in *every* setting, by *every* person, *every* day. Clinical expertise is no longer enough. Today, great caregivers see patients as unique individuals with lives, families, and goals, instead of as illnesses or injuries that need medical attention. In this regard, the best healthcare providers

- deliver the right resources at the right time;
- demonstrate behaviors that show they understand individual needs;
- involve patients and their families in care and decision making;
- ensure a culture of transparency, acknowledging that consumers are better informed than ever and have more resources at their disposal to make smart healthcare decisions; and
- appreciate that the competition in today's marketplace means that only organizations that focus on the whole patient experience will make the cut.

To underscore this point, the *Futurescan* survey results indicate that 80 percent of executives expect that by 2021 healthcare consumers will compare their hospital's patient experience rating against those of other hospitals before deciding where to receive care.

Fundamentals of Change

The evolution of the patient experience is being driven by a number of key factors, specifically

- new delivery models,
- patient-centered care,
- changes in reimbursement, and
- consumerism.

New delivery models: We are entering a new era in which the patient experience will

About the Author

Christy Dempsey is the chief nursing officer for Press Ganey Associates, Inc., responsible for providing clinical guidance to help clients transform the patient experience. She leads the team in efforts to reduce patient suffering and develop compassionate and connected care across the continuum. Dempsey is a registered nurse with more than three decades of healthcare experience in nursing, perioperative and emergency services management, medical practice, supply chain and materials management, and physician–hospital collaboration. She speaks and publishes nationally and internationally on patient experience, patient flow, physician–hospital collaboration, and balancing cost and quality. She also serves as faculty for the Missouri State University Department of Nursing. Dempsey has master's degrees in both business and nursing and is certified in both perioperative nursing and executive nursing practice.

FUTURESCAN SURVEY RESULTS:
The Patient Experience

How likely is it that the following will be seen in **your hospital** by 2021?

Very Likely (%)	Somewhat Likely (%)	Somewhat Unlikely (%)	Very Unlikely (%)
33	46	17	3

The majority of your patients will have compared your patient experience ratings with those of other hospitals before choosing to receive services at your hospital.

Very Likely (%)	Somewhat Likely (%)	Somewhat Unlikely (%)	Very Unlikely (%)
51	38	9	2

Your hospital will partner with current or former competitors in population health initiatives.

Very Likely (%)	Somewhat Likely (%)	Somewhat Unlikely (%)	Very Unlikely (%)
42	42	14	3

At least 10 percent of your hospital's total possible reimbursement will depend on the achievement of Consumer Assessment of Healthcare Providers and Systems (CAHPS) scores in multiple areas of the hospital.

Very Likely (%)	Somewhat Likely (%)	Somewhat Unlikely (%)	Very Unlikely (%)
61	35	3	1

Your hospital will assign care teams made up of diverse professionals, rather than single individual contributors, to patients with some types of conditions.

Very Likely (%)	Somewhat Likely (%)	Somewhat Unlikely (%)	Very Unlikely (%)
23	45	27	5

Your hospital's leaders will measure organizational performance primarily using patient experience metrics.

Very Likely (%)	Somewhat Likely (%)	Somewhat Unlikely (%)	Very Unlikely (%)
54	41	5	◊

Your hospital's human resources strategy (staff training, rewards, and recognition) will be designed to emphasize positive patient experience outcomes.

Note: Percentages may not total to exactly 100% due to rounding.
◊ Less than 0.5%

The Patient Experience: What Practitioners Predict

Patients will consult patient experience ratings when choosing where to receive hospital care. Almost 80 percent of practitioners surveyed expect that by 2021 patients will compare their hospital's patient experience rating against those of other hospitals before choosing to come to their hospital for care.

continued on pg. 8

—continued from pg. 6
increasingly be associated with how consumers and payers define value. Value-based care will take on a broader context than just the number of discharges, surgeries, and procedures. The new equation will include clinical measures, patient experience metrics, readmissions, and hospital-acquired conditions, among other factors.

In light of this trend, patient experience will become even more important to hospital executives and boards. In fact, two-thirds of *Futurescan* survey respondents predict that by 2021 administrators will assess how hospitals and health systems are doing primarily using patient experience measures. Because the patient experience encompasses clinical, operational, cultural, and behavioral aspects of care, it must become the principal evaluation tool for organizational performance.

The evolving healthcare marketplace will also encourage more collaboration among providers. Research shows that the best outcomes are achieved by robust programs that deliver consistent results over time (Sternberg and Dougherty 2015). This requires high volumes of patients and the necessary resources

to optimize care. Because volume and resources are not possible for every healthcare organization, collaboration in the form of referrals to medical centers of excellence—including those that may have been competitors in the past—will become necessary.

Population health management, bundled reimbursement, and accountable care organizations will also necessitate this kind of joint effort. Indeed, providers may need to collaborate with the hospital down the street to provide the best care for a defined group of patients. Achieving high quality requires understanding the needs of people in these population groups, regardless of their health status.

Patient-centered care: Care teams focused on patients rather than on the convenience of healthcare organizations are key to improving the patient experience. The University of Texas MD Anderson Cancer Center's head and neck program in Houston is one example of an organization that aligns resources to provide better care. Instead of requiring patients to travel to multiple facilities, the program consolidates caregivers, testing, and treatments in one location

so that patients have access to the right interprofessional team at the right time in the right place. In addition to enhancing the patient experience, this approach provides greater efficiency for the organization and reduces the cost of care (Porter 2010).

Changes in reimbursement: Increasingly, provider payments are being tied to patient satisfaction measures. Hospital Consumer Assessment of Healthcare Providers and Systems (HCAHPS) scores already account for 30 percent of a hospital's value-based purchasing (VBP) score (Medicare.gov 2015). While VBP scoring may change in the future, 84 percent of *Futurescan* survey respondents believe that by 2021 at least 10 percent of their organization's total reimbursement for care will be linked to consumer assessment scores.

Just as HCAHPS has changed the way providers think about the inpatient hospital experience, so, too, will the expected implementation of similar consumer assessments for outpatient care redefine how the patient experience is measured (and reimbursed). For example, the rollout of emergency department (ED) scores, known as

continued from pg. 7

Competitors will cooperate on population health initiatives. The majority (89 percent) of survey respondents think their hospital will partner with current or former competitors to work on population health initiatives by 2021.

CAHPS scores will influence reimbursement. Most (84 percent) of those responding to the survey believe that by 2021 at least 10 percent of their hospital's total possible reimbursement for care will depend on the achievement of CAHPS scores in multiple areas of their hospital.

Hospitals will treat patients with certain conditions using care teams. Almost all survey respondents (more than 96 percent) agree that within the next five years their hospital will treat patients with some types

of conditions by assigning them care teams made up of diverse professionals, rather than single individual contributors.

Patient experience metrics will be used to evaluate organizational performance. About two-thirds (68 percent) of practitioners answering the survey predict that by 2021 senior leaders will assess their hospital's organizational performance primarily using patient experience metrics.

Staff development and rewards will emphasize positive patient experience outcomes. Almost all (95 percent) of those surveyed are in agreement that by 2021 their hospital's human resource strategy, including staff training, rewards, and recognition, will emphasize positive patient experience outcomes.

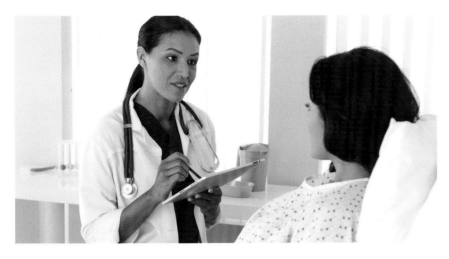

EDCAHPS, is certain to change how the patient experience is viewed in the ED. The proliferation of these surveys underscores the importance of the patient experience—clinically, operationally, culturally, and behaviorally.

Consumerism: A growing number of consumers are "shopping" for medical services by comparing prices and searching the Internet for patient ratings before choosing providers. To take control of their brand, healthcare organizations must accept and embrace this new age of transparency, understanding that complete and honest reporting of patient experience data is paramount to meeting patient needs. As healthcare pivots to value rather than volume, transparency will allow focused efforts aimed at improving outcomes as well as reputation (Glickman et al. 2010; Lee 2013).

Nearly all *Futurescan* survey respondents (96 percent) report that they commonly collect data that provide a complete view of the patient experience with their hospital. Many share the information with their communities to increase transparency and drive decision making. These pioneering organizations are transforming healthcare through consumer engagement.

Implications for Caregivers

Healthcare leaders need to acknowledge that patient loyalty is driven by perceptions. Patients' willingness to recommend or rate a provider more highly

than others is influenced, in part, by whether they believe doctors and nurses work effectively together to provide coordinated care.

Patients frequently find the healthcare system difficult, if not impossible, to navigate. On entering the hospital, many patients fear a loss of control and the risk that implies. They may be concerned that their care team does not seem to communicate, and they may feel frustrated by repeatedly being asked the same questions. They may wonder why tests are duplicated and information is not shared with them. When collaboration among caregivers is lacking, it demonstrates organizational dysfunction that may lead to adverse events and poor outcomes.

Engaging physicians, nurses, and other employees directly involved in patient care is critically important to optimizing the patient experience. Press Ganey research related to nurse engagement indicates that while nurses are generally engaged with their patients, those who are most engaged are not nurses at the bedside but rather nurses in administrative or support roles (Dempsey, Reilly, and Buhlman 2014).

Additionally, the data from Press Ganey research show that nurses are most engaged when they have been at a healthcare organization less than six months. Engagement then falls dramatically and does not begin to rise again until the nurse has been with the organization for more than ten years (Dempsey, Reilly, and Buhlman 2014).

Human resource strategies must focus on improving engagement and retention efforts with nurses in the intervening period to reduce the risk of experience and expertise walking out the door.

The average turnover rate for nurses in 2014 was 16.4 percent, according to the *2015 National Healthcare Retention & RN Staffing Report* (NSI Nursing Solutions 2015). The cost of turnover for a bedside nurse ranged from $36,900 to $57,300, leading to a loss of $6.2 million for an average hospital. Nursing turnover thus costs US hospitals billions of dollars each year.

The good news is that an engaged nurse is 87 percent less likely to leave an organization (Corporate Leadership Council 2004). Furthermore, engaged nurses are more likely to be satisfied with their jobs and think highly of the quality of care delivered at their hospital or health system. Positive correlations are also seen between nurse engagement and patient experience in terms of HCAHPS scores for prompt response to call lights and reductions in hospital-acquired conditions such as falls, pressure ulcers, and central line–associated bloodstream infections.

The connections between caregiver engagement and patient satisfaction are too strong to ignore. In fact, 95 percent of *Futurescan* survey respondents agree that staff development and rewards positively influence patient experience and clinical outcomes.

Role playing and simulations that allow caregivers to feel what patients feel and to receive immediate coaching is one way innovative healthcare organizations are showing their employees how to improve the patient experience. Renown Regional Medical Center in Reno, Nevada, provides an excellent example. Jeff Stout, vice president and chief nursing officer of the acute care division, says that as part of orientation new ED staff members are asked to report to the department. On arrival, they are directed to a waiting room where they must sit for four hours without being given any information. The employees are then taken to a treatment room where the curtain is closed, and, again, no information is shared. They are able to hear everything that happens on the other side of the curtain, including what others say about them, but still no information is provided. At the end of the day, a preceptor walks in and says, "This is what patients go through every day. Don't forget it."

The reality is that many caregivers have never been patients themselves.

This type of role playing is therefore critically important.

Conclusion
The patient experience is so much more than patient satisfaction. Reimbursement changes will require healthcare organizations to think about the patient experience in terms of meeting the unique needs of individuals and their

families and improving the value of care provided in every setting by every person. At the same time, consumers are choosing health services based on experience and clinical quality measures that are publicly reported. Clearly, understanding the totality of the patient experience will be paramount to remaining competitive in the healthcare marketplace of the future.

References

Corporate Leadership Council. 2004. *Driving Performance and Retention Through Employee Engagement*. Washington, DC: Corporate Executive Board.

Dempsey, C., B. Reilly, and N. Buhlman. 2014. "Improving the Patient Experience: Real-World Strategies for Engaging Nurses." *Journal of Nursing Administration* 44 (3): 142–51.

Glickman, S.W., W. Boulding, M. Manary, R. Staelin, R.J. Wolosin, E.M. Ohman, E.D. Peterson, and K.A. Schulman. 2010. "Patient Satisfaction and Its Relationship with Clinical Quality and Inpatient Mortality in Acute Myocardial Infarction." *Circulation: Cardiovascular Quality Outcomes* 3 (2): 188–95.

Lee, J. 2013. "Wal-Mart, Lowe's to Offer Employees Leg Up on Knee and Hip Work—at Certain Systems." *Modern Healthcare*. Published October 8. www.modernhealthcare.com/article/20131008/NEWS/310089966.

Medicare.gov. 2015. "The Total Performance Score Information." Accessed November 18. www.medicare.gov/hospitalcompare/data/total-performance-scores.html.

NSI Nursing Solutions. 2015. *National Healthcare Retention & RN Staffing Report*. East Petersburg, PA: NSI Nursing Solutions, Inc.

Porter, M.E. 2010. "What Is Value in Health Care?" *New England Journal of Medicine* 363 (26): 2477–81.

Sternberg, S., and G. Dougherty. 2015. "Risks Are High at Low-Volume Hospitals." *US News and World Report*. Published May 18. www.usnews.com/news/articles/2015/05/18/risks-are-high-at-low-volume-hospitals.

The Coming "Kitty Hawk Moment" in Healthcare Strategic Capital

by Michael Irwin

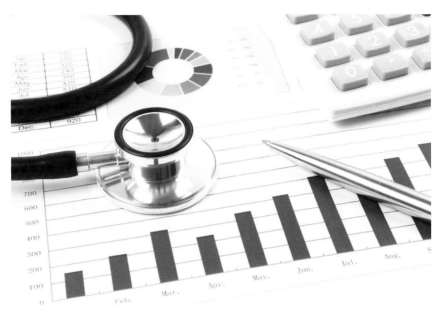

In his wonderful eponymous book on the Wright brothers, author David McCullough (2015) provides an insight on a critical moment in the history of flight when Wilbur and Orville began experimenting with manned aircraft at Kitty Hawk, North Carolina, in 1900. Previously, all would-be aviators (including the bike-mechanic brothers themselves) believed the key to flying was building a more powerful engine. However, the brothers quickly realized that one factor was even more important than power: *control*. Only with this realization did they begin to make the progress that led to their ultimate success.

A similar moment appears to be at hand for healthcare organizations as they transition from a hospital-centric business model to one based on fully integrated care, population health management, and increased consumerism. While executives have rightfully focused on the operational imperatives associated with these changes, they have paid much less attention to their implications for their capital strategy. As a result, even a number of today's most forward-thinking health systems may be sitting on top of a capital structure more suited to an earlier age.

In the coming years, many healthcare leaders will reexamine their assumptions about how to finance and manage the risk of a dramatically different enterprise. Like the Wright brothers, most of them will find that looking beyond conventional wisdom is the key to success.

The Past and Present of Healthcare Capital

To better understand how the current capital structure of hospitals evolved, realize that healthcare's traditional business model is really that of a utility. Most of today's hospitals developed in a world where certificate-of-need laws provided meaningful barriers to entry and cost-based reimbursement ensured a thin but stable level of cash flow. Not surprisingly, the result was an industry characterized by a higher level of debt relative to assets than would be acceptable in most sectors. Since the primary physical asset of most hospitals was an expensive "big-box" facility, prudent financial managers sought to match those assets with debt amortized over a 25- or 30-year term.

Cost-based reimbursement actually encouraged highly leveraged balance sheets by providing higher payment to hospitals with larger depreciation and interest expenses. In keeping with this approach, the favored financing vehicle was the tax-exempt municipal bond. While the capital structures and spending priorities for most providers have

About the Author

Michael Irwin is a director in the not-for-profit healthcare group at Citi, a global financial services firm based in New York City. He has served as an investment banker and trusted adviser to many prestigious academic medical centers and healthcare systems over a 30-year career. He assists these clients with all aspects of their capital financing activities, including public and private debt offerings, as well as providing advisory services in connection with strategic transactions. Irwin received his bachelor's degree in economics from Providence College and his master of business administration degree from Pace University, where he received the Wall Street Journal Student Achievement Award for Finance.

Capital Strategies

How likely is it that the following will be seen in **your hospital** by 2021?

Very Likely (%)	Somewhat Likely (%)	Somewhat Unlikely (%)	Very Unlikely (%)
15	35	36	14

At least 10 percent of your hospital's strategic capital will come from equity and quasi-equity sources, such as joint ventures and/or minority (i.e., noncontrolling) investments.

9	34	39	17

Your hospital or health system will reevaluate the cost/benefit of maintaining high credit ratings and accept a lower credit rating largely to permit greater strategic flexibility.

ACHE

16	40	30	13

SHSMD

20	52	23	5

Both

17	43	29	11

The proportion of your hospital's investment portfolio invested in strategic opportunities not directly related to your core businesses (such as potentially disruptive technologies and/or services), which take advantage of institutional knowledge and resources, will be at least 10 percent higher than it is now.

8	21	42	29

At least half of the debt capital for your hospital will come from taxable financing sources.

Note: Percentages may not total to exactly 100% due to rounding.

Capital Strategies: What Practitioners Predict

Practitioners are divided about future sources of capital. Half (50 percent) of practitioners answering the survey predict that by 2021 at least 10 percent of their hospital's strategic capital will come from equity and quasi-equity sources, such as joint ventures and/or noncontrolling (i.e., minority) investments. The other half consider this unlikely.

continued on pg. 13

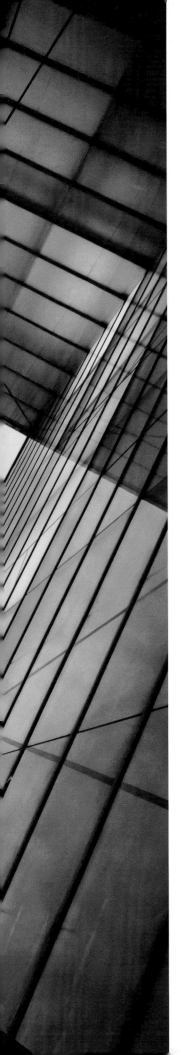

—continued from pg. 11

changed, there is still strong evidence of the continued use of this model.

The five-year financial plan for many organizations may still include major inpatient projects, but the focus is increasingly on expanding ambulatory and physician networks and adding information technology. The importance of growth is well understood, and the industry as a whole is seeing an accelerating level of horizontal provider consolidation as well as myriad vertical initiatives.

For some health systems, the cost of expansion has been the assumption of legacy liabilities and debt from past hospital-centric acquisitions that could hamper their ability to invest in transformation, especially when they continue to be challenged by shrinking margins. In recognition of this conundrum, a growing number of executives are embracing joint ventures. With so much to do on so many fronts and a keen appreciation for the need to move quickly, the opportunity to collaborate—often with a for-profit company—provides valuable operational capabilities and capital resources. Through joint ventures, organizations can quickly achieve the objectives of scale without assuming the same debt burden as going it alone.

This, however, is where organizational strategy collides with capital strategy. By moving into new territories with new partners, many not-for-profit health systems have discovered that their historical funding vehicle of choice—the tax-exempt bond—no longer works as well as it once did.

Tax-exempt bonds impose limitations that often conflict with new strategic directions. At issue are legal restrictions that prevent the use of this type of financing for projects beyond their strict charitable purposes. As providers continue to merge and enter into joint ventures with physicians or for-profit partners, meeting the administrative burden of tax law becomes more difficult. For example, a new electronic health record system that will be available to doctors not employed by a hospital is generally excluded from tax-exempt funding. The same is true of an ambulatory surgery center operated in partnership with a for-profit orthopedic group. Even outsourcing the revenue cycle function to a for-profit company could trigger a remediation requirement such as accelerated debt repayment.

These issues are causing many healthcare leaders to rethink, as Wilbur and Orville Wright did, "power versus control" in their strategic capital decisions. Increasingly, large

continued from pg. 12

Practitioners are divided about the trade-off between strategic flexibility and maintaining high credit ratings. Slightly more than half (57 percent) of practitioners surveyed do not believe that within the next five years their hospital will accept a lower credit rating to permit greater strategic flexibility. However, almost half (43 percent) predict this will happen in their hospital.

Practitioners are divided about investment in strategic opportunities. Slightly more than half (56 percent) of ACHE members responding to the survey predict an increase of at least 10 percent in the proportion of their hospital's investment portfolio invested in strategic initiatives that are not related to their core businesses and that take advantage of institutional knowledge and resources (e.g., potentially disruptive technologies and/or services). A much larger proportion (72 percent) of respondents receiving the survey from SHSMD believe that within the next five years the fraction of their hospital's investment portfolios devoted to such strategic investments will increase by at least 10 percent.

Most debt capital will come from nontaxable sources. Only 29 percent of practitioners surveyed believe that by 2021 half or more of their hospital's debt capital will come from taxable sources.

organizations are finding that the flexibility provided by taxable corporate debt creates an attractive alternative to tax-exempt bonds.

Multiple Advantages

First, a misconception needs to be cleared up. Some healthcare executives assume that taxable bonds carry a much higher borrowing cost than tax-exempt debt does. In reality, the cost differential between the two options is marginal at best, thanks to the extremely affordable interest rates that have prevailed since 2008.

Corporate bonds are priced off US Treasury bond rates, which have remained at historically low levels since the beginning of the Great Recession. Often over the past five years, Treasury rates have actually been lower than the Municipal Market Data (MMD) index on which tax-exempt bonds are based (Exhibit 2.1). Still, because not-for-profit healthcare organizations are not yet fully appreciated by corporate investors, the "quality spread" (the interest premium above the index rate)

has been wider in the corporate market than in the municipal market. As a result, borrowing costs for taxable and tax-exempt funding have been comparable over the past several years. Many experts believe this trend of using taxable debt will continue and could accelerate in the future even if interest rates rise.

In short, market conditions since the credit crisis have provided an amazing opportunity for providers to transition to taxable debt solutions and take advantage of the following benefits:

- Taxable debt offers a ready and flexible currency for pursuing growth. Several health systems have raised significant "war chests" in the taxable market. Unlike traditional tax-exempt bonds, this corporate debt can be used to fund acquisitions in any state.
- Taxable funding can help organizations deal with problematic debt assumed through acquisitions. For example, acquired assets may raise questions about past exempt use or have outstanding bonds with unacceptable covenants.

Other assets may be ineligible for tax-exempt refunding. In all cases, the taxable financing option provides significantly more flexibility.

Prepare for the New Market

Recent years have seen dramatic increases in taxable funding by not-for-profit health systems (Exhibit 2.1), yet the advantages are often underappreciated. That may be why the majority of executives who responded to the *Futurescan* survey do not believe this strategy will play a significant role in their future debt offerings. Regardless, healthcare executives should fully understand how taxable financing can benefit their organizations. Here are a few recommendations.

Understand investors. The corporate-sector investor base is wide. It includes both domestic and international investors, and it encompasses insurance companies, hedge and pension funds, and others that may not be active in the municipal market. To understand these investors better, consider attending at least

Exhibit 2.1

Not-for-Profit Healthcare Taxable Bond Issuance, 2011–2015

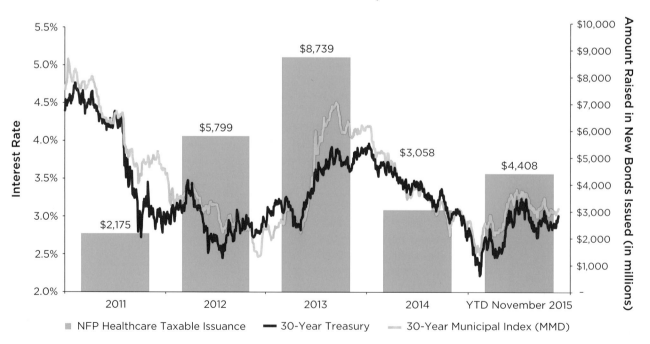

Source: Securities Data Corporation, Bloomberg. Reprinted with permission.
Notes: Data include publicly offered bonds only and exclude private and direct placements. NFP = not-for-profit.

one of the industry conferences sponsored by major Wall Street firms each year. Investor conferences provide an invaluable opportunity not only to learn about the taxable debt market but also to investigate potential joint venture partners.

Understand the market's sensitivities. Corporate investors are much more sensitive to size than are their municipal counterparts, in terms of both the profile of the borrower (probably best measured by top-line revenue) and the amount being raised (potentially hundreds of millions of dollars per offering). In both cases, larger is better. Accordingly, larger healthcare organizations will have an advantage in the corporate debt market.

Watch ratings implications. A strong credit profile is essential for all borrowers. Nonetheless, corporate investors have long afforded capital access at reasonable rates to for-profit hospital management companies even when their credit ratings were well below those of their not-for-profit counterparts. Time will tell whether these investors will adequately reward not-for-profit borrowers for their AA and A credit ratings with a meaningfully lower borrowing cost.

Help educate the market. Many corporate investors need to better understand the transformation underway in healthcare. Organizations that take the time to educate these investors about the opportunity of clinical integration will narrow the credit quality gap and reduce future borrowing costs.

Know the options. In addition to the public markets, many healthcare organizations are finding that taxable private placements—principally debt placed directly with insurance companies—are an attractive option. These deals can be accomplished in less time, without ratings, and without public disclosure—and at rates comparable to those achieved in a public offering. The ability to negotiate repayment terms directly with investors provides added flexibility to structure amortization around existing debt service requirements.

Learn from for-profit healthcare. Although their mission, vision, and values remain paramount, not-for-profit health systems should consider attaching greater importance to performance indicators emphasized by their for-profit counterparts. The debt-to-cash-flow ratio, for example, may provide a better tool for strategic capital planning than debt-to-assets or total capitalization. Focusing on this indicator can lead to greater alignment between debt levels and current and future earnings. For some systems, a plan to deleverage the balance sheet might be a logical outcome of this exercise.

Toward Transformational Investment

As part of a shift in thinking about strategic capital, healthcare organizations should reevaluate several assumptions about key capital decisions:

- In evaluating potential joint ventures, executives should explore new ways of thinking about control. Identify the things that are critical—such as quality and brand—and pursue how to secure these contractually but not necessarily through holding a majority interest. Particularly in joint ventures with physicians, health systems should consider shared governance and risk and not insist on majority control. The primary focus must be on strategic alignment, immediate downstream financial benefits, and future cash flow—whether above or below the operating income line.

- As leaders reevaluate their business model, they should remain open to dramatic conclusions. In the hospitality industry, a similar exercise several years ago led to a divestiture of large real estate holdings. Could this happen in the healthcare sector? It already has in long-term care and senior housing as the result of investments by real estate investment trusts (REITs). Several healthcare REITs have shown interest in expanding into acute care, as evidenced by recent major transactions. For some organizations, real estate divestiture could provide a means to reduce debt levels or redeploy assets into new strategic investments without bloating their balance sheets.

- Executives should consider making strategic investments in areas that could disrupt their current business model, including technology and service companies that are complementary to the healthcare industry. Such investment decisions could allow organizations to benefit by being both an accelerator of new ideas and an investor in them.

Discipline and Innovation

The bottom line is that dramatic changes in the healthcare business model will soon trigger corresponding changes in the industry's debt and capital structure. In a time of transformation, healthcare leaders should be disciplined, innovative, and open to new ways of addressing capital issues. Organizations that move beyond the conventional wisdom to develop a creative strategic capital plan will have the best chance of managing the complex transitions that will dominate healthcare in the years ahead.

Reference
McCullough, D. 2015. *The Wright Brothers.* New York: Simon & Schuster.

Leading Change: A Guide for the Perplexed

by Todd D. Jick, PhD

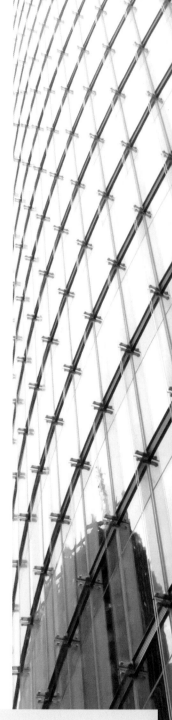

As an expert in leading change, I have often asked executive groups this question: What industry is most stable and least likely to experience transformation? The evolution of the answers over time has been telling.

In the 1990s, executives would name insurance, energy and gas, government, pharmaceuticals, or the post office. It was hard to argue with the responses. At the time these were all stable industries, with captive or loyal customers, that could focus the majority of their attention on finding efficiencies while growing steadily.

By the 2000s, however, the answers to the question had markedly changed. At one session, there was silence. Finally, someone jokingly said, "dry cleaners, funeral homes, and dairy farms." Immediately, there was debate about even these businesses given the greening pressures on dry cleaners, the consolidation of funeral homes, and the disappearance of the small farmer.

Today, as a result, I ask executive groups a different question: Do you feel you have reached the saturation point in dealing with and driving change in your organization? Again, the answers are telling. Typically, about half of the leaders reply that they are already saturated, overwhelmed, and under water. The other half, while not yet saturated, describe as many as five change-related challenges on their plates.

Clearly, all industries are experiencing significant transformations. The winners will be the executives who can best manage and lead their organization through a world of continuous change driven by technology, competition, globalization, customer pressure, government regulation, or shareholder activism.

The future may be more trying for some industries than for others. A 2014 poll of managers across all sectors found that the highest level of perceived at-or-near-change saturation was in retail (90 percent), telecommunications (83 percent), and healthcare (81 percent) (Creasey and Taylor 2014). The transitions in healthcare are formidable in the face of government intervention and regulations, fundamental business model shifts, complex stakeholder interests, medical advances, and consumerism—and the responses to the *Futurescan* survey indicate the challenges will only get more difficult in the years ahead.

Trends in Change Management

Change management is only about 75 years old, dating back to the work of Kurt Lewin (1943), a social psychologist who created the "force field analysis" concept. According to

About the Author
Todd D. Jick, PhD, is on the faculty of Columbia Business School in New York City. Previously, he was a professor at the Harvard Business School and a visiting professor in organizational behavior–human resource management at INSEAD and the London Business School. He received his master's degree and doctorate in organizational behavior from Cornell University. Dr. Jick is a leading expert in leadership and organizational change. His textbook *Managing Change* (McGraw-Hill, 2010) has been the leading offering in the field for the past 15 years, and his cases have been among the top sellers in case clearinghouses. He is also coauthor of *The Boundaryless Organization* (Jossey-Bass, 2002), which won the Accord Group Executive Leadership best business book of the year award in 2003. He has been actively involved in executive education, off-site and conference facilitation, and consulting in the areas of leadership, strategic planning, executive coaching, organizational change and transformation, values-based management, service management, and human resources management. Jick is president of Global Leadership Services, Inc., a consulting firm specializing in leadership and executive development support.

FUTURESCAN SURVEY RESULTS:
Leading the Change from Volume to Value

How likely is it that the following will be seen in **your hospital** by 2021?

Very Likely (%)	Somewhat Likely (%)	Somewhat Unlikely (%)	Very Unlikely (%)
43	33	18	6

Less than 60 percent of your hospital's total reimbursements will come from fee-for-service arrangements.

Very Likely (%)	Somewhat Likely (%)	Somewhat Unlikely (%)	Very Unlikely (%)
35	51	12	2

More than 10 percent of your hospital or health system's commercially insured reimbursements will flow through a bundled payment model.

Very Likely (%)	Somewhat Likely (%)	Somewhat Unlikely (%)	Very Unlikely (%)
29	29	26	16

Your hospital or health system will merge with, acquire, or be acquired by another hospital or health system.

Very Likely (%)	Somewhat Likely (%)	Somewhat Unlikely (%)	Very Unlikely (%)
11	48	32	9

Open or newly created senior leadership positions in your hospital will be filled by candidates from outside of the healthcare industry at least in part to tap expertise in effective consumer-centric strategies.

Very Likely (%)	Somewhat Likely (%)	Somewhat Unlikely (%)	Very Unlikely (%)
38	48	13	2

Your hospital or health system will have made a strategic multiyear investment totaling at least 5 percent of annual expenditures over that period in new solutions that support the transition from volume-based payments to value-based payments.

Very Likely (%)	Somewhat Likely (%)	Somewhat Unlikely (%)	Very Unlikely (%)
60	36	4	1

Your hospital will collect data that will yield a complete and actionable view of your patient's experience with your services.

Note: Percentages may not total to exactly 100% due to rounding.

Leading the Change from Volume to Value: What Practitioners Predict

Hospitals will move away from fee-for-service arrangements. Three-quarters (76 percent) of survey respondents expect that by 2021 less than 60 percent of their hospital's total reimbursement will come from fee-for-service arrangements.

continued on pg. 18

—continued from pg. 16

Lewin, the task of a leader is to increase the potency of the forces for change and decrease the effect of the restraining forces (Jick 1991). His work was a useful building block for what has become a blossoming, full-fledged field over the past decade—perhaps most clearly symbolized by the founding in 2011 of the Association of Change Management Professionals (ACMP), which has created certification standards and holds many conferences where ideas and best practices are exchanged. The ACMP has more than 2,000 members, including a large contingent from healthcare.

Another promising trend is the emergence of change management "centers of excellence." Notable companies that have such centers include Nike, IBM, Verizon, Blue Cross, and Caterpillar. These centers provide expert resources to organizations facing challenges as a result of technology, mergers, downsizing, and reorganization.

Courses taught in MBA programs on change have also expanded in number and popularity, and textbooks and case studies on the topic are widely available (e.g., Jick and Peiperl 2010). Executives are increasingly taking professional development classes on leading change, especially as more companies measure and evaluate administrators on this competency.

Despite all the progress, success rates remain underwhelming. A recent McKinsey survey found that 70 percent of change management efforts fail because of employee resistance or poor management support (Ewenstein, Smith, and Sologar 2015). That is a slight improvement over previous research studies, which indicated a 75 percent failure rate. The sobering conclusion is that leading transformation requires a rare mix of skill, discipline, and commitment.

Why is change so hard to manage? Organizations are facing conditions that are difficult to cope with individually let alone in aggregate, such as volatility, uncertainty, complexity, and ambiguity (the so-called VUCA world of the future). Success will be defined by the ability to

- chart a different course;
- navigate turbulence;
- adapt quickly to changing circumstances; and
- deal with opposition to a new direction, work process, or company structure.

Leaders will be challenged to step up their game in ways that will test their intellect, patience, and resilience. They will need to be agile in their thinking and create organizations that are flexible. The work ahead is perhaps akin to pioneering, because no one has trod this path before. There is no manual or road map. However, guidelines and principles are available that can help executives adjust to and even leverage the VUCA world. Let's examine what that world is predicted to be and its implications for healthcare professionals.

Implications for Leaders

Given the emergence of VUCA, the *Futurescan* survey findings point to three challenges executives will need to address over the next five years: managing business model transitions, overseeing organizational consolidation, and upgrading leadership capabilities.

continued from pg. 17

More hospital reimbursements will be part of a bundled payment arrangement. Eighty-six percent of survey respondents predict that by 2021 more than 10 percent of their hospital's commercially insured reimbursements will flow through a bundled payment model.

Practitioners are divided about mergers and acquisitions. A little more than half (58 percent) of survey respondents think their hospital or health system will merge with, acquire, or be acquired by another hospital or health system within the next five years. The rest (42 percent) consider this unlikely.

Hospitals will hire senior leaders from outside of healthcare to become more consumer-centric. Almost 60 percent of practitioners answering the survey believe that within the next five years open or newly created senior leadership positions in their hospital will be filled by candidates not currently in the healthcare field, at least in part to tap expertise in effective consumer-centric strategies.

Hospitals will invest in the transition from volume to value. The majority (almost 86 percent) of survey respondents agree that over the next five years their hospital will make a strategic multiyear investment totaling at least 5 percent of the hospital's annual expenditures in new solutions that support the transition from volume- to value-based payments.

Hospitals will collect complete and actionable patient experience data. Almost all survey respondents (96 percent) are in agreement that by 2021 their hospital will collect data that yield a complete and actionable view of the patient experience with their hospital's services.

Managing business model transitions:
The survey results confirm that the healthcare business model is shifting, so leaders must figure out how to optimize reimbursement in the new environment. Doing so will likely involve new stakeholders, new relationships with current stakeholders, new partners, and perhaps new skills. Providers recognize that the historic system of payments and profits is being transformed. Nobody is surprised anymore when a news story appears titled "Startups Vie to Build an Uber for Heath Care" (Beck 2015).

Clearly, rack rates and other revenue conventions are things of the past, and creative options for generating income are the new focus. This part of the VUCA world requires a different form of leadership. A new book describes it as "stragility"—continually sensing and evaluating shifts in a business model and making necessary modifications (Auster and Hillenbrand 2016). Conventional strategy processes will not succeed against nimble competitors in an evolving landscape; isolating uncertainties, undertaking scenario planning, and identifying key triggers of needed change are required for tomorrow's strategy (Toner et al. 2015).

Leaders have to be open-minded and willing to transition more rapidly to new models and platforms. This is no easy task. It requires dialogue, exposure to diverse views, experimentation, and humility to recognize that "what got us here may not get us there."

Overseeing organizational consolidation: More than half of the respondents to this year's *Futurescan* survey expect their organization to merge or be acquired in the next five years. In 2015 alone, consolidation activity among pharmaceutical and healthcare providers reached an estimated record level of $4.58 trillion (Mattioli and Strumpf 2015). These daunting figures underscore the importance of investing the time and resources necessary to find the right partner. It is never too early in the courtship to examine organizational culture differences, technology challenges, personnel strengths and weaknesses, and other potential challenges.

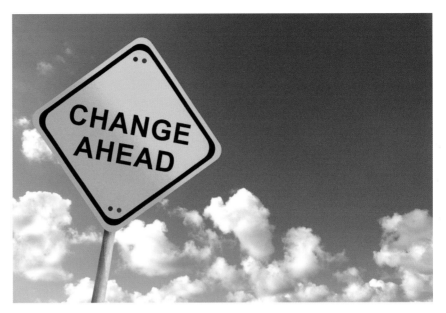

Well-developed best practices in merger and acquisition management and leadership are available to help with the process (e.g., Mirvis and Marks 2003).

Upgrading leadership capabilities:
Who is most qualified to steer organizations through the turbulent VUCA times that lie ahead? According to *Futurescan* respondents, almost 60 percent of vacant hospital and health system leadership positions will be filled by executives from outside healthcare. Such has been the recent trend in the private sector, although the number remains a minority at 30 percent (Palmquist 2013). Outsiders are typically chosen in turnaround situations and in times of business model transformation because they often have more experience in leading change management. Insiders are considered less likely to shake things up. In the end, organizations are still statistically more likely to promote from within, but the growing percentage of outsiders suggests that the skills needed for the future may best be found in executives from other industries.

The leader of complex change will also have to engage with a wider set of internal and external stakeholders. The ability to influence others, to engage in negotiations with partners, and to prioritize stakeholders in terms of importance and impact will all be part of the new equation. Leaders will have to be visible, transparent, and increasingly accessible. Finally, for change initiatives to be successful, executives will need to recognize that they cannot lead alone. Indeed, in a rapidly changing world one can excel only through distributed leadership, in which multiple voices are tapped and collaboration and dialogue become essential to solving complex challenges of business models and their execution.

Ready for the Future? A Note of Optimism

The capacity for change is both a survival method and a competitive advantage. A commitment to build this capacity and to manage the volume of changes both simultaneously and sequentially is vital. But this challenge is not for the faint of heart.

Change is difficult, and it is not going to get any easier in most industries, especially healthcare. However, a recent IBM study confirms what I have noticed over 35 years of studying and instituting organizational change: The success rate increases to 80 percent in the hands of "change masters" and diminishes to 20 percent in the hands of "change novices" (Jorgenson, Bruehl, and Franke 2014). In other words, by having skilled change leaders, by devoting resources to centers of excellence, by committing to spend the time needed to involve people in change, and by exercising the flexibility and agility required in the fast-paced VUCA world, there is hope and there is reward. Surely, increasing the likelihood of achieving the mission of healthcare is worth the effort. Buckle up, but equip yourself for the ride.

References

Auster, E.R., and L. Hillenbrand. 2016. *Stragility: Excelling at Strategic Changes.* Toronto, ON: University of Toronto Press.

Beck, M. 2015. "Startups Vie to Build an Uber for Health Care." *Wall Street Journal,* August 11.

Creasey, T., and T. Taylor. 2014. *2014 Best Practices in Change Management.* Loveland, CO: Prosci Inc.

Ewenstein, B., W. Smith, and A. Sologar. 2015. "Changing Change Management." McKinsey & Company. Published July. www.mckinsey.com/insights/leading_in_the_21st_century/changing_change_management.

Jick, T.D. 1991. "Implementing Change." Harvard Business School case 9-491-114. Boston: Harvard Business School Publishing.

Jick, T.D., and M. Peiperl. 2010. *Managing Change: Cases and Concepts*, 3rd ed. New York: McGraw-Hill.

Jorgenson, H.H., O. Bruehl, and N. Franke. 2014. *Making Change Work . . . While the Work Keeps Changing: How Change Architects Lead and Manage Organizational Change*. IBM Global Business Services report. Somers, NY: IBM Corporation.

Lewin, K. 1943. "Defining the 'Field' at a Given Time." *Psychological Review* 50 (3): 292–310.

Mattioli, D., and D. Strumpf. 2015. "Merger Activity Is on Pace for Record." *Wall Street Journal,* August 11.

Mirvis, P.H., and M.L. Marks. 2003. *Managing the Merger: Making It Work.* Washington, DC: Beard Books.

Palmquist, M. 2013. "Research Perspectives on the New CEO." *Strategy and Business*. Published May 28. www.strategy-business.com/article/00185.

Toner, M., N. Ojha, P. de Paepe, and M. Simoes de Melo. 2015. "A Strategy for Thriving in Uncertainty." Bain & Company brief. Published August 12. www.bain.com/publications/articles/a-strategy-for-thriving-in-uncertainty.aspx.

Rise of the Accelerators: The Growth of Health System–Based Investment and Innovation Programs

by Ezra Mehlman

The past five years have been a time of great uncertainty for healthcare executives. The migration to new payment methodologies, the compression of fee-for-service rates, an influx of newly insured patients, and a dizzying array of legislative "carrots" and "sticks" have combined to form a perfect storm, rendering the status quo untenable. In this frenzied environment of dwindling margins and regulatory confusion, health systems have begun to find new growth opportunities by experimenting with investment and innovation programs, or accelerators.

This article evaluates the models accessible to health systems that are interested in launching such programs. Throughout, it draws on the perspectives of executives from several organizations that are at the forefront of innovation. For example, Rich Roth, chief strategic innovation officer for Dignity Health, notes, "Providers all have a responsibility to continually innovate to offer better value to patients. Dignity

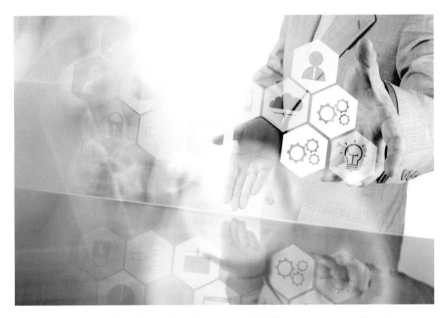

Health's focus is to blend our clinical expertise with the expertise that novel entrepreneurial companies have to offer. We want to help scale innovations to truly benefit patients with demonstrated results." Equipped with the insights of these experts, we can identify a set of implications for other healthcare leaders.

Health systems generally seek to achieve four principal goals when considering whether to undertake investment and innovation opportunities (Exhibit 4.1):

1. **Financial returns:** Many organizations establish investment

About the Author

Ezra Mehlman is a vice president at Health Enterprise Partners (HEP), a healthcare information technology and services–focused growth equity fund whose capital comes from some of the largest hospital systems, healthcare insurance companies, and pharmaceutical firms in the United States. By partnering with leading healthcare organizations, HEP is afforded a unique window into the rapidly evolving priorities of those responsible for shaping the direction of the industry. In turn, HEP is able to identify innovative companies that map to the executive playbook. Previously, Mehlman spent several years as a strategy consultant focused exclusively on the provider market, first at The Advisory Board Company and then at Booz Allen Hamilton. He currently serves as a director of InDemand Interpreting, CenterPointe Behavioral Health System, Applied Pathways and as a board observer of Evariant. He holds an adjunct appointment at Columbia University, where he co-teaches the healthcare investment and entrepreneurship course. Mehlman holds a master of business administration degree from Columbia University and a bachelor's degree in history, cum laude, from Washington University in St. Louis.

FUTURESCAN SURVEY RESULTS:
The Rise of Accelerators

An **IT accelerator**, sometimes referred to as an "incubator" or "venture lab," is a program that promotes the growth of private technology companies. This program may encompass the commercialization of internal ideas, technology pilot programs, direct investments in early-stage companies, investments in venture capital or private equity funds, and partnerships with other like-minded institutions to support the exchange of innovation.

How likely is it that the following will be seen in **your hospital** by 2021?

Very Likely (%)	Somewhat Likely (%)	Somewhat Unlikely (%)		Very Unlikely (%)

ACHE

8	21	35	36

SHSMD

23	26	34	17

Both

11	22	35	31

Your hospital will be invested in a healthcare venture capital or healthcare private equity fund.

14	30	32	24

Your hospital will have a healthcare IT accelerator in place.

11	20	34	35

Your hospital will have direct investments in healthcare IT companies.

8	12	30	50

Your hospital will acquire or develop one or more healthcare IT companies.

Note: Percentages may not total to exactly 100% due to rounding.

The Rise of Accelerators: What Practitioners Predict

Hospitals are not likely to invest in venture capital or healthcare private equity funds. Overall, about two-thirds (66 percent) of practitioners responding to the survey consider it unlikely that their hospital will invest in a healthcare venture capital or private equity fund within the next five years. However, respondents receiving the survey from ACHE and SHSMD differed in their responses. A higher proportion of SHSMD respondents (49 percent) than ACHE respondents (29 percent) predict that their hospital will invest in such funds.

continued on pg. 23

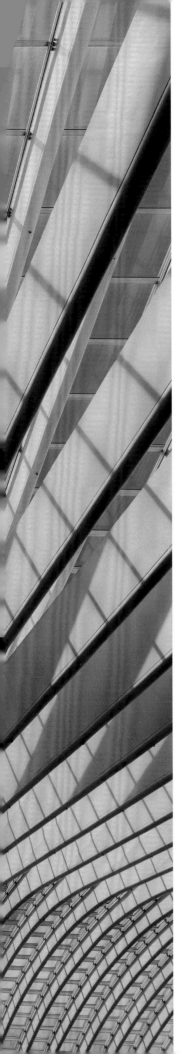

—continued from pg. 21

initiatives to drive financial returns. By taking equity stakes in early- and growth-stage companies and growing revenue through customer relationships, health systems can generate new sources of income that are not subject to the reimbursement pressures affecting the core business of delivering medical care.

2. **Operations improvement:** Innovation programs offer providers a means to identify a pipeline of promising companies that can help them upgrade operations, reduce medical costs, improve outcomes, and expand access to care.

3. **Brand enhancement:** Investment programs can serve as vehicles to enhance brand integrity in an increasingly competitive landscape through differentiation and expansion of market reach.

4. **Foster innovation:** Perhaps most significant, commercializing new ideas enables organizations to cultivate an innovation-focused culture.

Elaborating on these points, Tom Thornton, executive vice president of North Shore Ventures, says, "Our mission is to identify and invest in novel technologies and business models that have the potential to generate revenue, improve patient care, and advance North Shore's growth and the future of our industry. To do this, we define innovation broadly—in terms of what it is, where it comes from, and who's responsible for it—and we embed innovation in every part of our business. Defining innovation so broadly has important benefits. The simple fact is that we create many more opportunities because we're looking in more places, and we're working with more partners."

Models of Health System–Based Investment and Innovation Programs

Depending on a given health system's risk appetite, resource commitment, and desired return, a variety of approaches are available (Exhibit 4.2):

- **Accelerator investments:** A number of third-party accelerators offer partner organizations access to—and a small equity stake in—a multitude of early-stage companies. A well-publicized investment in an internal accelerator program may confer branding benefits, in addition to providing interaction with other health systems that have made similar commitments.

- **Innovation centers:** Developing an in-house innovation center enables organizations to generate revenue from internal intellectual property (IP). Such a center may take the form of an internal accelerator, whereby new products are researched, developed, and launched using a health system's own resources. A successful center typically incorporates the following:
  - Mining mechanisms to identify ideas with commercial potential
  - Screening processes to filter the most compelling concepts
  - Matching components to pair prospective entrepreneurs with the staffing, financial, and clinical resources needed to bring ideas to market

- **Warrant deals:** Several organizations have developed warrant programs, in which

continued from pg. 22

Practitioners are divided about the prevalence of hospital-based IT accelerators. More than half (56 percent) of survey respondents do not believe that by 2021 their hospital will have an IT accelerator in place. A little less than half (44 percent) predict that their hospital will have an IT accelerator in place.

Most hospitals will not invest directly in healthcare IT companies. Sixty-nine percent of practitioners surveyed do not think their organization will invest directly in health IT companies within the next five years.

Most hospitals will not acquire or develop healthcare IT companies. Most (80 percent) of those responding to the survey do not believe their hospital will acquire or develop one or more healthcare IT companies by 2021.

Exhibit 4.1

Goals of Strategic Healthcare Investing

Financial Returns	Operations Improvement	Brand Enhancement	Foster Innovation
	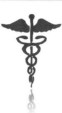	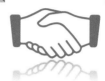	
Secure a favorable financial return by taking an equity stake in a company with which the system has a relationship	Leverage portfolio companies to solve the system's challenges	Create direct and indirect value via both brand extension and association with other market players	Provide a window into emerging innovations and gain a top-down look on emerging trends

the health system picks up an equity percentage in a company in conjunction with signing a commercial agreement. This approach provides executives with a low-risk means to share in the upside while minimizing the downside financial risk.

- **Fund investments:** This option offers the opportunity to invest in a portfolio of companies while not being tied to the fate of any single business. It also allows organizations to benefit from the due diligence and investment management resources of a fund, rather than assuming this burden themselves.

- **Direct investments:** Increasingly, health systems are making direct equity investments in healthcare information technology (IT) and service firms to leverage commercial relationships with these vendors. While representing the biggest possible financial return, direct investments also carry the greatest amount of risk because financial returns are linked to one company. Aaron Martin, senior vice president of strategy and innovation for Providence Health & Services, describes the experience of operating

a $150 million dedicated venture capital fund: "The fund is highly integrated into our innovation agenda and works closely with digital and innovation teams that are making large investments in software engineering and new consumer-health business models. We generally seek to make direct equity investments in early- to mid-stage businesses where Providence is committed to developing a strategic relationship. We believe that such investments strengthen our alignment with portfolio companies because we strive to help them hone more effective products and navigate the challenges of deploying technology in healthcare provider organizations."

- **Co-invest with sponsor:** By co-investing in healthcare companies alongside a fund, health systems can leverage the due diligence and deal execution resources of an institutional investor while gaining access to the equity upside that accompanies direct investments. These opportunities frequently take the form of an opening or an extension to an institutional funding round for a select "strategic" to join the syndicate. In conjunction with a co-investment,

health systems may implicitly or explicitly commit to pursuing a commercial relationship with the target company.

Of course, these models are not mutually exclusive. Sophisticated organizations will typically apply a multipronged strategy in operating an investment and innovation program—featuring, for example, internal IP commercialization alongside external investment activity.

Emblematic of this diversified approach is Intermountain Healthcare. Bert Zimmerli, the health system's chief financial officer, says, "We don't see innovation as optional. To deliver on the promise of helping people live the healthiest lives possible in an era of population health management, innovation is essential. In the past five years, we recognized the need to go beyond the status quo and begin implementing new programs to further liberate innovation from within. We also recognized that it takes dedicated capital to help ideas come to life, so we created an innovation fund to support these efforts now and in the years ahead. So far, the feedback from innovators is positive, generating a lot of goodwill with physicians and other caregivers in our ranks.

Exhibit 4.2

Universe of Investment Options and Their Trade-Offs

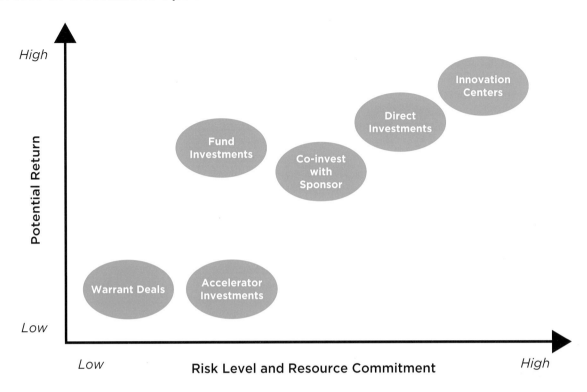

Intermountain has long held the view that innovation can lead to better care and lower costs. For example, we've partnered with wireless sensor companies to analyze patient data in new ways that have led to a sensor-based surgical ambulation program that is shortening lengths of stay and lowering readmissions for our patients."

Implications for Healthcare Leaders

The evolving landscape of innovation and investment programs has a number of implications for healthcare leaders.

A new paradigm of health systems working with early-stage companies has emerged. While the features of innovation and investment programs vary widely across organizations, all mandate a new mode of working with early-stage companies. The prohibitively long sales cycles these businesses customarily face when selling in a healthcare setting represent a major deterrent for entrepreneurs attempting to penetrate this

segment. In many ways, the barriers to sales represent barriers to innovation. Breaking down these obstacles will require a systematic method of screening companies against organizational objectives and identifying the appropriate business unit champions to help them reach decision makers. This relationship needs to work both ways; health systems should be rewarded for the effort and risk associated with supporting early-stage businesses.

An internal resource commitment is essential. Undertaking an investment and innovation program in earnest requires both executive sponsorship and a dedicated financial and personnel commitment. If the intention is to transform a health system's core business model for the future, then executives would be well served to treat the program as a priority. Rich Adcock, executive vice president of Sanford Health, offers the following perspective: "Sanford Frontiers is designed to 'improve the human condition' through the development of new

devices and therapeutics that improve quality and create nontraditional revenue. By providing resources for our physicians and scientists, we pave the path for their entrepreneurial pursuits. In less than three years, Frontiers supported the development of a fully licensed medical device, moving from the concept stages through the patent process and clinical trials to taking the product to market. Frontiers also supports the development of consumer health products and programs. For example, the organization's weight loss program has grown to include 25 stores in ten states serving more than 20,000 members. Over a short period, our investment in innovation has paid dividends, both monetarily and in a culture shift among our professional teams."

Innovation program structure depends on goals and risk appetite. With a multitude of available options, healthcare leaders must prioritize and decide which investments are most appropriate for their organization's risk appetite and return goals. Structuring warrant deals with companies or investing in an external accelerator presents a reasonably low risk of losing capital, but these approaches do not offer substantial upside potential. Conversely, making direct investments in companies or rolling out an internal IP commercialization effort comes with higher levels of both financial risk and return. Exhibit 4.3 outlines a number of factors executives should consider in launching their programs.

Revenue diversification is the name of the game. In many ways, the rise of health system investment and innovation programs has paralleled the rollout of risk-based payment models. Healthcare reform has galvanized executives to think more critically about margin enhancement strategies. While some providers have been laser focused on doing anything they can to maximize profitability under the fee-for-service system, others understand that surviving in a new world, in which health systems are assuming significant financial risk for a patient's treatment, will require new ideas, products, and sources of revenue.

Conclusion

A market scan shows widespread agreement among leaders that innovation is no longer optional for health systems. The question thus becomes how to develop and implement an investment and innovation strategy that meets an organization's distinctive financial, strategic, and marketing goals while staying within internal resource constraints. This article provides a high-level evaluation of the universe of options accessible to providers and shares the perspectives of several nationally renowned experts in the field.

While the *Futurescan* survey data provide some indication of where executive attitudes lie—33 percent predict they will invest in a venture capital or private equity fund by 2021, and nearly half (44 percent) believe they will have an IT accelerator in place in that time frame—the right choice for any given organization depends on the trade-off between risk and return. Although few organizations have "cracked the code" on strategic investing and innovation, studying the best practices of those that have done so is an important exercise for any health system leader who stands on the precipice of launching an internal investment and innovation program.

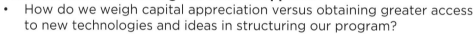

Exhibit 4.3

Considerations in Launching Investment Programs

What are our investment goals and risk appetite?
- How do we weigh capital appreciation versus obtaining greater access to new technologies and ideas in structuring our program?
- What is our investment horizon?
- Are we comfortable taking on greater downside risk in exchange for a higher potential return?

How are we sourcing and evaluating new opportunities?
- Is our current pipeline sufficient?
- How do we best mine internal intellectual capital?
- Are we deploying internal resources efficiently and appropriately?

How will the program be governed and staffed?
- What will the metrics be for defining program success, and how will reporting be coordinated?
- Who will maintain ultimate oversight over the program?
- Will we repurpose existing team members, or will we recruit and build a full internal investment team?

How can we differentiate our program?
- With many intelligent investors chasing the same companies, how can we provide something uniquely valuable?
- How do we drive commercial value for prospective portfolio companies internally?

The Future of Healthcare for Veterans: Partnerships

by Robert A. McDonald

Shannan Brown, a young peer support specialist at the Department of Veterans Affairs (VA) Medical Center in Manchester, New Hampshire, has partnered with a local horse farm where she now brings women veterans for brief retreats.

For two relaxing days, these veterans—many of them coping with military sexual trauma and post-traumatic stress disorder (PTSD)—can ride horses; tend to the goats, chickens, and other animals that live on the farm; or just go for a quiet walk in the woods. Most important, they get to spend time with fellow women veterans who understand what they are going through. The emotional benefits of this experience are nothing less than phenomenal.

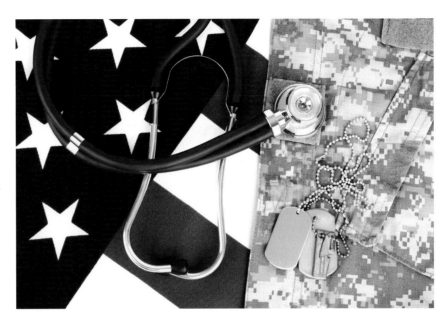

The Power of Partnerships

As VA embarks on perhaps the most sweeping transformation in its 85-year history, a major component of that transformation will involve what Brown is doing so well in New Hampshire: creating partnerships.

To that end, VA is striving to improve its partnerships with nonprofit, community-based groups and more effectively collaborate with federal, state, and local agencies that can address veterans' healthcare, housing, and employment needs. VA can only meet the considerable challenges it faces in these areas if it nurtures and strengthens the partnerships it has already formed and continuously works to establish new ones.

For example, in the spring of 2014 an all-day wellness retreat was held at VA's Burlington Lakeside Clinic in Vermont. About 30 women veterans attended the event, which featured nearly 20 free workshops and demonstrations, including "Building Resilience Through Self-Compassion," "Healthy Eating for Women," and "The Philosophy Behind Acupuncture," to name a few. All workshops were offered by local practitioners who volunteered their time because they care.

About the Author

Robert A. McDonald was nominated by President Obama to serve as the eighth secretary of the US Department of Veterans Affairs (VA) and was confirmed by the US Senate on July 29, 2014. Prior to joining VA, Secretary McDonald was chairman, president, and chief executive officer of Procter & Gamble Company (P&G). Under his leadership, P&G significantly recalibrated its product portfolio; expanded its marketing footprint, adding nearly one billion people to its global customer base; and grew the firm's organic sales by an average of 3 percent per year. During his tenure, P&G was widely recognized for its leader development prowess. In 2012, *Chief Executive* magazine named it the best company for developing leader talent.

An Army veteran, Secretary McDonald served with the 82nd Airborne Division; completed jungle, arctic, and desert warfare training; and earned the Ranger tab, the Expert Infantryman Badge, and Senior Parachutist wings. On leaving military service, Secretary McDonald was awarded the Meritorious Service Medal.

FUTURESCAN SURVEY RESULTS:
Reengineering

How likely is it that the following will be seen in **your hospital** by 2021?

Very Likely (%)	Somewhat Likely (%)	Somewhat Unlikely (%)	Very Unlikely (%)

Very Likely	Somewhat Likely	Somewhat Unlikely	Very Unlikely
92		7	◊ 0

Patients in your hospital will be able to access their electronic health records online.

69	30	1	0

Patients in your hospital will demand a greater role in the planning of their treatment.

38	50	11	1

Twenty-five percent of persons requiring care for chronic conditions or rehabilitative care will receive it remotely using technologies depending on transmission of data from physical sensors.

54	41	5	0

Your hospital will use software products to track the use of resources and project their utilization.

64	32	3	1

At least one target for a population health metric will be established through collaboration between your healthcare system or hospital executives and leaders in local public health/nonprofit agencies.

26	57	16	1

The per capita rates for Ambulatory Care Sensitive Conditions hospitalizations will be reduced by 20 percent.

Note: Percentages may not total to exactly 100% due to rounding.
◊ Less than 0.5%

Reengineering: What Practitioners Predict

Patients will be able to access their health records online. Virtually all practitioners surveyed (99 percent) agree that their hospital's patients will be able to access their electronic healthcare records online within the next five years.

continued on pg. 29

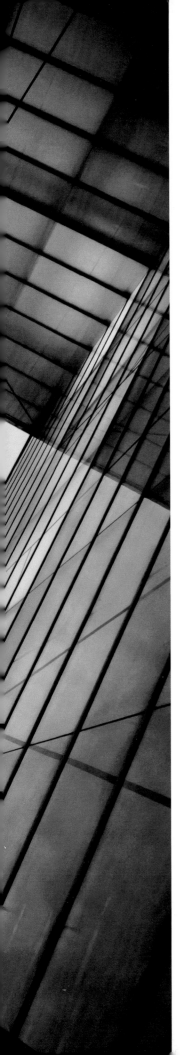

—continued from pg. 27

The retreat was organized by Dr. Laura Gibson, director of behavioral health at VA's Burlington Lakeside Clinic and clinical associate professor of psychology at the University of Vermont, who said she was "moved by how many community professionals volunteered to introduce these techniques to the women." With mind–body approaches gaining traction among the general population for pain management, improved sleep and immune function, stress and blood pressure reduction, and overall health and well-being, Dr. Gibson noted, "It's not surprising that these approaches are sought after by service members and veterans as well."

Through this type of community involvement, VA is increasingly using complementary and integrative therapies as a means of supplementing conventional behavioral health and pain management programs. More and more, the department is turning to yoga, acupuncture, music therapy, equine therapy, and other modalities as it focuses on treating the "whole veteran" and reducing patients' dependence on opioid prescriptions as their primary coping mechanism.

Another example of the power of partnerships is the fight against homelessness among veterans. VA has joined forces with hundreds of community partners throughout the country who have made it their business to ensure that every veteran who wants a roof over his or her head has one.

Consider the good work of Kelly Estle, who for six years served as a social worker at VA's outpatient clinic in Mobile, Alabama. Estle routinely worked with her local Veterans of Foreign Wars, American Legion, Salvation Army, and two other nonprofit groups—Waterfront Rescue Mission and the Fifteen Place day shelter—to get homeless veterans off the streets. And what she accomplished in Mobile is something VA is trying to replicate elsewhere. Last summer, for instance, marked the launch of a national program to help the roughly 50,000 unemployed, homeless veterans find jobs with employers in their communities.

Without question, VA is what it is today because of partnerships. The department recognizes that it does not have all the answers or all the means necessary to meet the needs of the country's veterans, so it is engaging the public

continued from pg. 28

Patients will participate more in planning their treatment. Virtually all survey respondents (99 percent) agree that by 2021 their hospital's patients will demand a greater role in the planning of their treatment.

Care will be delivered remotely using data gathered from physical sensors. Most (nearly 88 percent) of practitioners surveyed predict that by 2021 at least 25 percent of persons requiring care for chronic conditions or rehabilitative care will receive it from their hospital remotely, using technologies that gather patient data from physical sensors.

Hospitals will use software to track and project resource utilization. Nearly all survey respondents (95 percent) believe that by 2021 their hospital will use software to track and project the utilization of hospital resources.

Hospitals will establish targets for population health metrics in collaboration with local public agencies. Almost all (96 percent) of those answering the survey agree that within the next five years their hospital's or health system's executives will establish at least one target metric for population health in collaboration with leaders of local public health or nonprofit agencies.

Rates for Ambulatory Care-Sensitive Conditions (ACSCs) will be reduced. Most (83 percent) of those responding to the survey predict that by 2021 the per capita rates for ACSC admissions to their hospital will be reduced by 20 percent.

and private sectors and academia like never before.

VA's first foray outside government was in 1946, when it teamed up with premier medical and health science schools to deliver care for the 16 million troops and 670,000 casualties who were demobilized after World War II. Today, VA partners with nearly 2,000 academic and research institutions and spends more than $650 million annually on medical and nursing school alliances that include some of the top universities in the country, such as Harvard and Stanford.

Since becoming VA secretary in July 2014, I have spent a lot of time on the road visiting VA facilities and the organizations the department works with across the nation. Everywhere I go, I see community involvement and collaboration:

- In April 2015, I was in Palo Alto, California, where I toured the Defenders Lodge, funded by Lee and Penny Anderson and the PenFed Foundation, where veterans and their caregivers can stay for free while being treated at the Palo Alto VA Health Care System.
- In March 2015, I visited Colorado for VA's annual Winter Sports Clinic, sponsored by Disabled American Veterans and a host of corporate donors, including Ford, Samsung, Prudential, and many others.
- In January 2015, I went to Chicago for a roundtable forum sponsored by City Colleges of Chicago, the Utility Workers Union of America, and a local utility on an innovative training program to get veterans working in the natural gas industry.
- In October 2014, I was in Kansas City, Missouri, for a World Series game dedicated to veterans. Before the game, I was shown what had been an old, empty building that was renovated and brought back to life as a VA hospital annex through the generosity of the Kansas City Royals, the Bank of America, and Major League Baseball.

The point is, plenty of opportunities exist for foundations, corporations, and individuals to help out with projects they can put their name on and say, "We did this for America's veterans." A perfect example is a nationwide initiative introduced in 2015 called a Summer of Service, in which VA is spurring local engagement and encouraging citizens to volunteer their time to help veterans. Imagine what could be accomplished if this kind of involvement began taking root in every community throughout the United States.

The Power of Preparation

Make no mistake—this "all hands on deck" approach will become increasingly critical as VA prepares for a challenge that has been in the making for some time: the rapidly growing population of aging veterans. Although the total number of veterans is actually declining, the number needing assistance from VA is on the rise because of the Vietnam War. In 1975, only about 2 million veterans were older than 65; by 2017 there will be almost 10 million.

Here is a sobering statistic: In just ten years, the number of people aged 65 and older with Alzheimer's disease is expected to jump by 40 percent (Richardson et al. 2015). An increasing number of those will be veterans because traumatic brain injuries or PTSD has made them twice as likely to develop dementia. To provide aging veterans with the care they deserve, VA must become better trained and equipped to deal with their physical and mental health problems.

VA also needs to bolster the emotional and financial support it provides to the legions of caregivers who are housing, feeding, and nurturing veterans. And, most important of all, VA must tap into the talent, expertise, and experience of those in the community who have dedicated years to learning about the health issues facing older adults.

The Power of Prevention

Did you know that from 2001 to 2011, according to the Centers for Disease Control and Prevention (CDC 2013), diagnoses of diabetes rose 62 percent in the United States—from 12.9 million to 20.9 million cases? Heart disease remains the country's leading cause of death, claiming the lives of more than 600,000 people (23.5 percent of the total) in 2013 (CDC 2015a). And 35 percent of US adults are obese (CDC 2015b). We spend more per capita on healthcare than does any other industrialized nation in the world, yet our average life expectancy is no better than that in countries that spend far less.

Clearly, providers need to redesign how care is delivered by shifting the focus from treating disease to maintaining and improving health. Many healthcare organizations understand this dynamic and have committed to the Institute for Healthcare Improvement's Triple Aim of better care, lower cost, and better health.

VA has unique opportunities to make a difference in the health of veterans. With the guidance of its partners in the community, the department is continuously searching for ways to assist veterans in making the right lifestyle decisions, including

- developing positive relationships,
- avoiding smoking and excessive use of alcohol,
- eating the right kind of foods,
- using mind–body techniques to manage stress, and
- exercising regularly.

By encouraging veterans to make the right lifestyle choices, VA can help them lower their risk for heart disease, diabetes, cancer, drug abuse, and other disorders.

The Power of Prediction

Partnerships will continue to be indispensable as VA explores a new frontier that may revolutionize its approach to medical care: genomics. The department is working on applying the potential of genetic mapping to develop safer, more effective treatments based on new knowledge about the role of genes in health and disease.

In 2011, VA launched its Million Veteran Program (MVP)—a partnership with veteran volunteers to learn more about how genes affect health. MVP is establishing one of the largest databases of genetic, military exposure, lifestyle, and health information for use in medical research. By identifying gene–health connections, MVP stands to significantly advance the screening, diagnosis, and prognosis for diseases while pointing the way toward more effective, personalized therapies. As providers get better at predicting the risk of certain conditions, the need for individuals to take a proactive, holistic approach to their health will become even more critical.

With an expected enrollment of 1 million veterans over the next five to seven years, MVP is already the largest database of its kind in the United States. But VA is not doing this important work alone. Bright minds throughout the world, in both the private and public sectors, are collaborating with the department to unlock the enormous potential of genomics.

Conclusion

The VA and providers across the nation are all on this journey together, because caring for veterans is a responsibility too complex and important to be tackled by a few organizations or government agencies. It is an obligation that can be fulfilled only by leveraging the power of partnerships. As Winston Churchill once stated, "If we are together nothing is impossible. If we are divided all will fail."

Acknowledgment

VA Deputy Secretary Sloan Gibson contributed to this article.

References

Centers for Disease Control and Prevention (CDC). 2015a. "Leading Causes of Death." Updated September 30. www.cdc.gov/nchs/fastats/leading-causes-of-death.htm.

———. 2015b. "Obesity and Overweight." Updated September 30. www.cdc.gov/nchs/fastats/obesity-overweight.htm.

———. 2013. "Number (in Millions) of Civilian, Noninstitutionalized Persons with Diagnosed Diabetes, United States, 1980–2011." Updated March 28. www.cdc.gov/diabetes/statistics/prev/national/figpersons.htm.

Richardson, P., D. Luzzatto, C. Hatcher, and S. Day. 2015. "Coming Crisis in Veterans Care." *Virginian-Pilot*, May 31.

Promoting Health: The One Alternative to Healthcare Rationing

by Michael F. Roizen, MD, and Olivia Delia

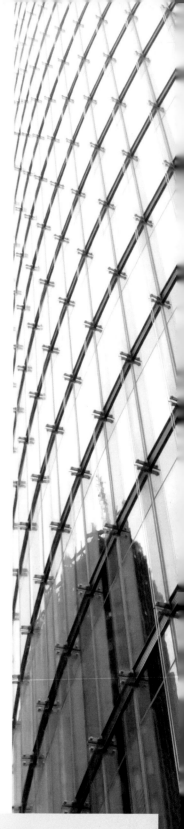

Healthcare in the United States is like food: When Americans are hungry, they want to eat something soon, and they want it to be good. Healthcare is the same: When patients have medical needs, they want to receive high-quality treatment as quickly as possible.

But that is where the similarity ends. Most people understand that there is a limit to how much they can eat (notice I said "most people," not "everyone"). However, the amount of healthcare Americans consume has been growing dramatically (Åkesson et al. 2014).

Most of the heightened demand is due to the increased prevalence of chronic disease, because we still

- use too much tobacco;
- eat too much inexpensive, addicting, and unhealthy food—250 or more calories a day more per person than in 1978–1983 (Gregg et al. 2014);
- are much less physically active than in 1990 (Vuori, Lavie, and Blair 2013); and
- experience excessive stress that we do not manage well.

Right now, 10 percent of Americans aged 47 or older develop a chronic disease each year. As a result, 97 percent of those enrolling in Medicare have unmanaged or undermanaged health problems. And currently, more than 80 percent of the nation's $2.5 trillion health spend goes to chronic disease management (Daviglus et al. 1998, 2005; Moses et al. 2013). At the top of the list are lifestyle-induced conditions that take the lives of more than seven in ten Americans, such as type 2 diabetes, dementia, cancer, osteoarthritis, heart disease, and stroke.

This influx of chronic disease has played a major role in declining prosperity and rising income inequality in our country (and in many others). Since 1997, every penny of increased wages for US workers has gone to the cost of medical care and medical insurance (Hancock 2012).

Unfortunately, the long-term trends look even worse. Between 1974 and 2014, the number of type 2 diabetics in the United States increased from 3.2 million to 29 million (Exhibit 6.1). Diabetes care now represents nearly 10 percent of healthcare expenditures—and between 1.5 and 2 percent of the gross national product (GNP). Experts predict that by 2050, 120 million to 180 million Americans will have diabetes—a six- to tenfold increase in a total US population that is projected to grow only 30 percent during that time (Bernstein et al. 2014; Ezzati and Riboli 2013; Gregg et al. 2014). With no new therapies, and assuming the average age of those treated remains constant (unlikely, since they will probably be older), caring for these individuals will account for 10 to 15 percent of the GNP. That's not 15 percent of healthcare spending, but 15 percent of the total US economy!

The same pattern can be seen in hip and knee replacement surgery (Exhibit 6.2), dementia care, post–heart attack care, post-stroke care, and post-cancer care. If current trends continue, by 2050 the amount of money the nation

About the Authors

Michael F. Roizen, MD, is the chief wellness officer at Cleveland Clinic. He graduated from the University of California, San Francisco, School of Medicine and performed his residency in medicine at Harvard's Beth Israel Hospital. He is certified by both the American Board of Internal Medicine and the American Board of Anesthesiology. Dr. Roizen is a *New York Times* best-selling author (four times at #1 and eight times overall) and a frequent guest on television news and talk shows. He still practices internal medicine.

Olivia Delia is a graduate of Williams College and a first-year medical student at the Perelman School of Medicine at the University of Pennsylvania. She was a science journalism intern with Dr. Roizen in 2014–2015.

FUTURESCAN SURVEY RESULTS:
Promoting Health

How likely is it that the following will be seen in your hospital's area by 2021?

Very Likely (%)		Somewhat Likely (%)	Somewhat Unlikely (%)	Very Unlikely (%)
47		42	9	1

Most insured patients will belong to health plans that pay substantial cash incentives (or reduce insurance premiums substantially) to beneficiaries for meeting certain health targets (e.g., healthy measurements in blood pressure, LDL cholesterol, fasting blood sugar, waist size, or absence of tobacco toxins.)

27	48		22	3

Most people will monitor their levels of stress with their phones or wearable devices.

36	41		19	4

Twenty-five percent of the population in your area will receive care from an ACO that is focused on population health.

Note: Percentages may not total to exactly 100% due to rounding.

Promoting Health: What Practitioners Predict

Most patients will receive cash incentives for meeting health targets. Most (89 percent) of those answering the survey anticipate that within the next five years most of their hospital's insured patients will belong to health plans that will substantially reduce insurance premiums for, or pay substantial cash incentives to, patients who meet certain health targets. These health targets include healthy measurements in blood pressure, LDL cholesterol, fasting blood sugar, waist size, and absence of tobacco toxins.

Most people will use phones or wearable devices to monitor stress. Three-quarters (75 percent) of survey respondents predict that by 2021 people in their hospital's area will monitor their stress levels using their mobile phones or wearable devices.

At least a quarter of the population in hospital service areas will receive care from an accountable care organization (ACO). More than three-quarters (77 percent) of survey respondents believe that by 2021 at least 25 percent of the population in their hospital's area will receive care from an ACO focused on population health.

Exhibit 6.1

Prevalence of Type 2 Diabetes in the United States

Year	Type 2 Diabetics	Total Population	Prevalence
1974	3.2 million	211 million	20/1,000
1983	4.6 million	235 million	24/1,000
1994	6.8 million	260 million	30/1,000
2004	15.0 million	292 million	55/1,000
2014	29.0 million	320 million	91/1,000
2050 (predicted)	120–180 million	430 million	279–418/1,000

Exhibit 6.2

Prevalence of Total Joint Arthroplasty in the United States

Year	Hip/Knee Arthroplasties	Total Population	Prevalence
1974	0.067 million	211 million	0.3/1,000
1990	0.327 million	235 million	1.4/1,000
1999	0.425 million	260 million	1.6/1,000
2000	0.441 million	292 million	1.5/1,000
2006	0.675 million	292 million	2.3/1,000
2010	1.050 million	320 million	3.3/1,000
2050 (predicted)	6.330 million	430 million	14.7/1,000

—continued from pg. 32
spends on treating chronic conditions in these six areas will consume nearly the entire GNP.

Back to the food analogy: No matter how much you like salmon burgers (notice I did not say "cheeseburgers"), you cannot eat 48 of them a day. The same is true of healthcare: The aforementioned spending increases are not realistic. America will have to either cut back on expenses or ration care.

A Proven Path to Outcomes-Based Wellness

Fortunately, another path is emerging. Under the leadership of Toby Cosgrove, MD, Cleveland Clinic has developed an effective new approach to employee wellness. If expanded to all populations, I believe it could achieve dramatic improvements in individual health and

meaningful cost reduction for the US healthcare system.

The approach is based on several large studies that demonstrate the importance of achieving normal measures in the following key metrics: low-density lipoprotein (LDL) cholesterol, blood pressure, blood sugar, waist-to-height ratio, stress management, and tobacco toxins (Exhibit 6.3). Cleveland Clinic calls them "the six normals." According to the literature, people who reach the six normals—with or without medication—reduce their subsequent chronic disease by 80 to 90 percent over 10- to 30-year periods (Åkesson et al. 2014; Chomistek et al. 2015; Daviglus et al. 2005, 2004; Stampfer et al. 2000; Willis et al. 2012).

But how do you motivate people to change their lifestyle? Cleveland Clinic explored many options before finding one that delivers major health benefits.

It is a thoughtfully structured, outcomes-based wellness strategy that not only prevents but actually reverses disease. In the process, it increases productivity, elevates morale, and produces savings for both employers and employees.

Cleveland Clinic found that five steps are essential to success:

1. Change the culture. The organization knew it could continue to lead in healthcare only if it stopped the influx of chronic disease. The financial case was clear: In 2005, healthcare costs for its 43,000 employees and 38,000 dependents had been increasing 9.5 percent per year. Based on projected growth, these costs would exceed $400 million by 2016, leaving the clinic unable to invest in people and innovative programs or adjust to expected decreases in reimbursement.

Exhibit 6.3

The "Six Normals" That Reduce the Risk of Chronic Disease by 80 Percent or More

Measure	Normal Range
Blood pressure	<140/90
LDL (bad) cholesterol	<100
Waist-to-height ratio	<0.5
Blood sugar	<100
Nicotine	Zero use
Stress	Routine practice of stress management

Starting in late 2005, Dr. Cosgrove began talking about these issues to all clinic caregivers literally every month. He presented the financial case, but he also emphasized the human case for reducing chronic disease. His strong leadership was critical to ingraining wellness into the organizational culture.

2. Change the incentive strategy. Early on, Cleveland Clinic tried offering small incentives (less than $400 per year) for healthy behaviors. It also emphasized process choices, such as undergoing a health risk assessment or walking 6,000 steps a day for 20 days each month. Unfortunately, this approach did not move the needle. Employees who were already healthy collected the dollars, those with incipient chronic disease progressed, and people with established chronic disease did not alter their lifestyle choices.

The needle moved dramatically only when we tied a substantial premium differential to biometric outcomes. Now when employees achieve the six normals and keep their immunizations up to date, they receive a premium reduction. The reduction was 20 percent in 2014 and is even higher now.

Cleveland Clinic has found that this significant savings incentive motivates healthy people to stay healthy. Individuals who are currently in a health improvement program to reach target levels are also eligible for a premium reduction. The few who will never be able to hit the six normals are allowed to qualify for an incentive through alternative goals established by their primary care physician.

3. Change the environment. Cleveland Clinic learned a lot when it banned smoking from its campuses in 2005. Previously, the organization reimbursed employees for up to 89 percent of the cost of its smoking cessation program. When it went smoke-free on all campuses, from Ohio to Abu Dhabi, the clinic made the program free. That day, four times as many people signed up for smoking cessation as had in the previous four years.

Essentially, Cleveland Clinic changed the environment by incentivizing employees to make healthy choices and by eliminating financial barriers to wellness. It also provides free on-site fitness clubs, weight loss memberships, and health coaching. The clinic's cafeterias have changed, too, removing all fryers and getting rid of sugared beverages from vending machines.

4. Establish care programs. Cleveland Clinic launched a number of free services to help staff with chronic conditions control and even reverse their disease. The programs are based in the clinic's primary care offices and are provided in person, via online consultations, and through shared medical appointments. Under the direction of physicians, nurses coordinate employees' care and educate them about food choices, stress management, and physical activity.

5. Encourage wellness. The clinic has also established free programs to assist healthy employees and those with incipient medical issues. The emphasis here is on creating fun opportunities through "health buddies," social media engagement, and e-coaching. Smartphone apps help participants maintain exercise goals and cope with stress.

The key to success is providing support. Poorly executed outcomes-based incentives can discriminate against the people who need help the most. If we simply charge higher premiums to employees who smoke or are overweight, we are only punishing them. But if we couple financial incentives with effective and free health programs, we empower individuals to overcome unhealthy behaviors.

The Result: A Clear Return on Investment

Cleveland Clinic's experience shows that outcomes-based wellness incentives work for both employers and employees. Here are some highlights:

- **The six normals:** Ninety-five percent of people who had six normals in 2009 maintained them through 2014. In addition, 63 percent of individuals with one or more out-of-range results have now achieved all of the measures or are working toward that goal.
- **Nicotine use:** Employee smoking rates have declined from 15.4 percent in 2004 to 5.3 percent in 2014.
- **Weight management:** Employees have collectively lost and kept off 450,000 pounds (as measured by their physicians) since 2011. Body mass index has declined 0.5 percent a year, whereas the national average is increasing 0.37 percent annually.

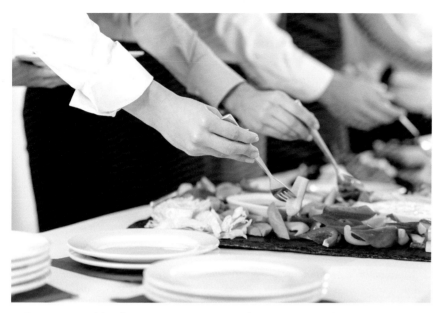

organizations in diverse industries establish similar programs. For example, Lafarge has realized estimated savings in excess of $200 million, Bon Secours's employee stress and engagement scores have improved by more than 40 percent, and Crum & Forster reports a first-year ROI of 341 percent.

Currently, only 3 to 4 percent of the population entering Medicare in the United States falls within range for all of Cleveland Clinic's health measures. Imagine the possibilities if hospitals and health systems joined the clinic in encouraging businesses, communities, and individuals across the country to embrace this proven approach to wellness. If only 65 percent of individuals achieved the six normals, the nation would save well over $600 billion in healthcare spending per year. Providers have the chance to lead the way like never before in decreasing the incidence of chronic disease, improving Americans' health, and reining in the spiraling cost of care. It is an historic opportunity we cannot afford to miss.

- **Cost savings:** The clinic estimates it saved at least $60 million in 2015 through improvements in employee wellness, a figure that has steadily increased every year since the launch of the initiative. This dramatic return on investment (ROI) does not even take into account the positive impact on absenteeism.

A Promising Future

The great news is that the six normals are exportable. In the past few years, Cleveland Clinic has helped several

References

Åkesson, A., S.C. Larsson, A. Discacciati, and A. Wolk. 2014. "Low-Risk Diet and Lifestyle Habits in the Primary Prevention of Myocardial Infarction in Men: A Population-Based Prospective Cohort Study." *Journal of the American College of Cardiology* 64 (13): 1299–306.

Bernstein, A.M., N. Rudd, G. Gendy, K. Moffett, J. Adams, S. Steele, and M. Frietchen. 2014. "Beliefs About Preventive Care, Individual Health, and Lifestyle Change Among Low-Income African American Women at Risk for Diabetes." *Holistic Nursing Practice* 28 (1): 24–30.

Chomistek, A.K., S.E. Chiuve, A.H. Eliassen, K.J. Mukamal, W.C. Willett, and E.B. Rimm. 2015. "Healthy Lifestyle in the Primordial Prevention of Cardiovascular Disease Among Young Women." *Journal of the American College of Cardiology* 65 (1): 43–51.

Daviglus M.L., K. Liu, P. Greenland, A.R. Dyer, D.B. Garside, L. Manheim, L.P. Lowe, M. Rodin, J. Lubitz, and J. Stamler. 1998. "Benefit of a Favorable Cardiovascular Risk-Factor Profile in Middle Age with Respect to Medicare Costs." *New England Journal of Medicine* 339 (16): 1122–29.

Daviglus, M.L., K. Liu, A. Pirzada, L.L. Yan, D.B. Garside, P. Greenland, L.M. Manheim, A.R. Dyer, R. Wang, J. Lubitz, W.G. Manning, J.F. Fries, and J. Stamler. 2005. "Cardiovascular Risk Profile Earlier in Life and Medicare Costs in the Last Year of Life." *Archives of Internal Medicine* 165 (9): 1028–34.

Daviglus, M.L., K. Liu, L.L. Yan, A. Pirzada, L. Manheim, W. Manning, D.B. Garside, R. Wang, A.R. Dyer, P. Greenland, and J. Stamler. 2004. "Relation of Body Mass Index in Young Adulthood and Middle Age to Medicare Expenditures in Older Age." *Journal of the American Medical Association* 292 (22): 2743–49.

Ezzati, M., and E. Riboli. 2013. "Behavioral and Dietary Risk Factors for Noncommunicable Diseases." *New England Journal of Medicine* 369 (10): 954–64.

Gregg, E.W., X. Zhuo, Y.J. Cheng, A.L. Albright, K.M. Venkat Narayan, and T.J. Thompson. 2014. "Trends in Lifetime Risk and Years of Life Lost Due to Diabetes in the USA, 1985–2011: A Modelling Study." *Lancet Diabetes & Endocrinology* 2 (11): 867–74.

Hancock, J. 2012. "Employer Health Costs Rise 4 Percent, Lowest Increase Since 1997." *Kaiser Health News*. Published November 14. http://khn.org/news/employer-health-costs-rise-4-percent-lowest-increase-since-1997/.

Moses, H., D.H. Matheson, E.R. Dorsey, B.P. George, D. Sadoff, and S. Yoshimura. 2013. "The Anatomy of Health Care in the United States." *Journal of the American Medical Association* 310 (18): 1947–63.

Stampfer, M.J., F.B. Hu, J.E. Manson, E.B. Rimm, and W.C. Willett. 2000. "Primary Prevention of Coronary Heart Disease in Women Through Diet and Lifestyle." *New England Journal of Medicine* 343 (1): 16–22.

Vuori, I.M., C.J. Lavie, and S.N. Blair. 2013. "Physical Activity Promotion in the Health Care System." *Mayo Clinic Proceedings* 88 (12): 1446–61.

Willis, B.L., A. Gao, D. Leonard, L.F. Defina, and J.D. Berry. 2012. "Midlife Fitness and the Development of Chronic Conditions in Later Life." *Archives of Internal Medicine* 172 (17): 1333–40.

Succeeding with New Payment Models

by Lee B. Sacks, MD, and Michael J. Randall, FACHE

The landscape of new healthcare payment models is changing rapidly. In the six months between the administration of the *Futurescan* survey and the publication of this article, several significant market developments have already taken place. More major insurers unveiled plans to merge, the Centers for Medicare & Medicaid Services (CMS) and state governments announced new programs, and payers and providers across the country continued to form innovative partnerships. Succeeding with new payment models has less to do with accurately predicting the future and more to do with creating a culture focused on cost and quality improvement, having the will to change, and fostering strong relationships with physicians and community organizations.

Forces Driving the Migration to Global Risk

Health economists, policy makers, and industry leaders often advise providers to accept risk in order to meaningfully improve costs. Until now, hospitals and health systems have largely resisted, but changing market forces are expected to accelerate the movement toward risk at a rate not seen since the 1990s.

Medicare managed care: An increasing number of health systems view Medicare managed care as a growth opportunity. About three-quarters (78 percent) of *Futurescan* survey participants predict that by 2021 at least 40 percent of their eligible patients will be covered through Medicare Advantage (MA) plans. Today, 30 percent of Medicare beneficiaries are enrolled in the plans, a figure that has tripled in the last ten years. MA penetration varies by state—from less than 1 percent in Alaska to 51 percent in Minnesota. Experts believe enrollment will grow 60 percent by 2024, in part as a result of increasing consumer awareness and comfort in selecting managed Medicare plans (Kaiser Family Foundation 2014).

Next Generation accountable care organization (ACO): Many health systems view the Next Generation ACO Model as a glide path to accepting global risk. The goal of the initiative, according to CMS (2015), is "to test whether strong financial incentives for ACOs, coupled with tools to support better patient engagement and care management, can improve health outcomes and lower expenditures."

Commercial insurance: The commercial insurance market is exerting equal pressure in propelling providers toward risk. About 11.4 million individuals were enrolled in health insurance through the public marketplace in 2015 (US Department of Health & Human Services 2015). Of these, 87 percent qualified for a federal subsidy that is likely to continue thanks to the US Supreme Court's decision on *King v. Burwell*.

About the Authors

Lee B. Sacks, MD, is executive vice president and chief medical officer for Advocate Health Care. He received an undergraduate degree from the University of Pennsylvania and a medical degree from the University of Illinois at Chicago. He completed a family practice residency at Advocate Lutheran General Hospital in Park Ridge, Illinois. He served as president of the Illinois Academy of Family Physicians and currently serves on the American Hospital Association's Committee on Clinical Leadership, which he chaired in 2015.

Michael J. Randall, FACHE, is chief administrative officer for Advocate Physician Partners. He received his master of healthcare administration degree from the University of North Carolina at Chapel Hill and his bachelor of science degree in movement science, with distinction, from the University of Michigan. He completed his administrative fellowship at NorthShore University Health System in Evanston, Illinois.

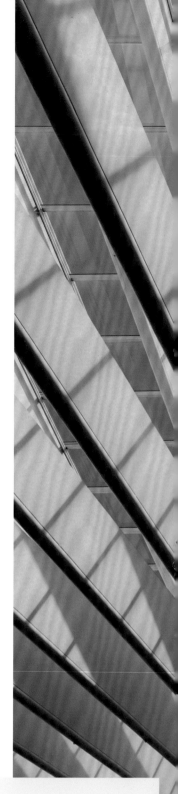

FUTURESCAN SURVEY RESULTS:
New Payment Models

How likely is it that the following will be seen in **your hospital** by 2021?

Very Likely (%)	Somewhat Likely (%)	Somewhat Unlikely (%)	Very Unlikely (%)
12	41	36	11

Your board or system officers, in your performance review, will evaluate you on your hospital's success in setting retail pricing.

| 27 | 51 | 20 | 2 |

More than 40 percent of your hospital's Medicare patients will be covered through Medicare Advantage.

| 56 | 34 | 8 | 1 |

The proportion of your hospital or health system's expenditures devoted to post-acute care capabilities (e.g., palliative care, hospice, or skilled nursing) will increase.

| 54 | 38 | 5 | 2 |

Your hospital or health system's investment in integrated behavioral health services (i.e., behavioral health services integrated with other care functions such as primary care, emergency department care, inpatient rounding, etc.) will increase.

ACHE

| 20 | 23 | 27 | 29 |

SHSMD

| 30 | 29 | 26 | 15 |

Both

| 23 | 24 | 27 | 26 |

Your hospital or health system will be licensed to sell its own health insurance products.

| 33 | 39 | 15 | 12 |

Your hospital or health system will have a cobranded product with an insurer.

Note: Percentages may not total to exactly 100% due to rounding.

continued on pg. 40

—continued from pg. 38

Private health exchanges: Perhaps an even bigger driver of change is the private health exchanges, which are soon expected to eclipse their public counterpart in total enrollment. Like the shift in retirement benefits from pensions to 401(k) plans, employers are beginning to move insurance coverage from a defined benefit to a defined contribution. As a result, the number of workers participating in private exchanges is expected to grow from the current 6 million to 40 million by 2018 (Birhanzel, Brown, and Tauber 2015).

Research shows that most consumers select health insurance coverage based on price. A survey of individuals enrolled in the Aon (2015) Active Health Exchange indicated that when choosing a coverage level, most based their choice on

- price (34 percent),
- similarity to their current plan (20 percent), or
- level of medical benefits (18 percent).

When choosing an insurance carrier, enrollees said they based their choice on

- the lowest cost for the selected coverage level (35 percent),
- network of doctors (23 percent), or
- past experience (11 percent).

Patients today are savvy customers. High deductibles are leading them to shop for the best price. Although *Futurescan* respondents are divided on whether retail pricing will become a performance metric for CEOs, providers still should evaluate their rates to ensure they are competitive with those of freestanding ambulatory centers and physicians for common procedures.

Reference pricing: Another cost savings tool expected to gain traction among businesses is reference pricing, which involves setting a cap on benefits for certain services offered by many providers with no discernible difference in quality. For example, a company may decide that it is willing to pay only $1,000 for a colonoscopy and that employees will be responsible for any additional expense above that amount. A 2014 survey by Aon Hewitt of 1,230 employers covering more than 10 million workers found

continued from pg. 39

New Payment Models: What Practitioners Predict

Practitioners are divided about whether hospital CEOs will be evaluated on their hospital's success in setting retail pricing. About half (53 percent) of practitioners responding to the survey predict that by 2021 hospital CEOs will be evaluated on their hospital's success in setting retail pricing. The other half (47 percent) do not believe successful retail pricing will be used as a metric to evaluate CEO performance.

A significant proportion of Medicare patients will be covered through Medicare Advantage. About three-quarters (almost 78 percent) of survey participants predict that by 2021 at least 40 percent of their hospital's patients eligible for Medicare will be covered through Medicare Advantage.

Hospitals will spend more on post-acute care capabilities. Almost all practitioners surveyed (more than 90 percent) predict that over the next five years their hospital or health system will increase the proportion of its expenditures devoted to post-acute care capabilities, such as palliative care, hospice, or skilled nursing.

Hospitals will increase their investment in integrated behavioral health services. Nearly all survey respondents (92 percent) believe their hospital or health system will increase its investment in behavioral health services that are integrated into other functions, such as primary care, emergency department services, and inpatient rounding, over the next five years.

Practitioners are divided about whether hospitals or health systems will sell their own health insurance products. Overall, roughly half (53 percent) of practitioners responding to the survey do not think their hospital or health system will be licensed to sell its own health insurance products by 2021. Almost as many (47 percent) predict their organization will sell such products. However, respondents receiving the survey from ACHE and SHSMD differed in their answers. More respondents receiving the survey from SHSMD (59 percent) than from ACHE (43 percent) believe their organization will be licensed to sell health insurance products.

Hospitals will have cobranded products with insurers. Almost three-quarters (72 percent) of survey respondents predict that by 2021 their hospital or health system will have a cobranded product with an insurer.

that 10 percent had already adopted reference pricing and that another 68 percent intended to do so in the next three to five years.

One way providers are responding is through bundled payments, in both commercial plans and Medicare. The rapid expansion of bundled-payment demonstration projects could mean that federal reimbursement based on this model is not far off. CMS has signaled that as early as 2016 bundled payments could replace diagnosis-related groups (DRGs) as the basis for reimbursement in some markets as part of the proposed Comprehensive Care for Joint Replacement Model.

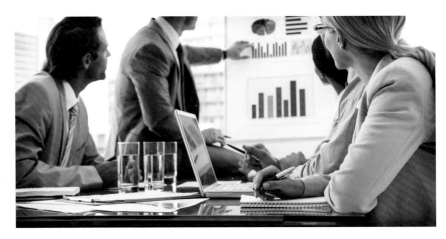

Post-acute care: As hospitals look for ways to lower costs and readmissions, post-acute care is beginning to get more attention. Almost all *Futurescan* executives surveyed (more than 90 percent) predict that by 2021 their organizations will increase the proportion of expenditures devoted to post-acute capabilities, such as palliative care, hospice, or skilled nursing.

An innovative strategy many health systems are exploring is contracting with independent skilled nursing facilities (SNFs). In this model, organizations have their advanced practice nurses, supported by appropriate physicians, rounding daily to manage care and outcomes and thereby reduce patient lengths of stay and acute care readmissions. At Advocate Health Care, for example, this approach has lowered the average length of stay by four days at an average savings of nearly $2,000 per case.

Additional areas of focus will include

- implementing remote patient monitoring for chronic disease management and
- combining remote monitoring and home visits to create a "hospital at home" as a substitute for inpatient admissions for conditions such as community-acquired pneumonia without respiratory distress, deep venous thrombosis, and upper urinary tract infections.

Integrated behavioral health services: As the healthcare environment changes, providers are exploring ways to use behavioral health services to reduce patient complications from chronic medical conditions. Progressive organizations are designing comanagement models of care and aligning their contracting approaches to support these efforts. Nearly all *Futurescan* survey respondents (92 percent) believe that in the next five years their organization will increase investment in behavioral health services that are integrated with other functions, such as primary care, emergency department services, and inpatient rounding.

Physicians and value-based care: In an effort to preserve reimbursement, more physicians are likely to approach local hospitals and health systems about participating in value-based care, through either bundled payments or ACOs. The Sustainable Growth Rate (SGR) fix injects another dose of motivation for physicians through the Alternative Payment Model value-based payment bonus methodology.

Strategies to Manage Global Risk

Providers are beginning to trade lower per unit prices for access to more lives. Borrowing another concept from the 1990s, organizations will form "high-performing networks." Unlike their "narrow networks" predecessor, high-performing networks will consist of premier-quality, low-cost providers selected on the basis of objective data.

Health systems and their physician partners should begin considering now whether they will build a network themselves or participate in an established network as a contracted party. They also should develop criteria (e.g., cost, patient experience, quality, patient-centered medical home adoption, meaningful use) to help them evaluate who will best position their organization for success. Almost three-quarters (72 percent) of *Futurescan* survey respondents predict that by 2021 their hospital or health system will have a cobranded product with an insurer.

Executives are divided about whether providers will offer their own health plans. Overall, nearly half (47 percent) of *Futurescan* respondents think their organization will be licensed to sell insurance products by 2021. By managing the full premium, providers have additional levers with which to influence caregiver and consumer behavior. As of 2013, about 12 percent of US hospitals had an equity stake in a health maintenance organization (Herman 2015). Most organizations start with Medicaid and their own associates. Depending on the market dynamics, provider-sponsored health plans may venture into Medicare Advantage and commercial offerings. Following are a few key questions to consider before developing an insurance product:

- Does creating a provider-sponsored health plan align with our mission and vision?
- Do we have the financial reserves to weather potential losses?
- Do we have a large enough membership to mitigate potential losses due to outliers?
- How will consumers respond?
- How will commercial payers respond?

Being both a payer and a provider can create friction in an organization. Interests may not always align. Success as a payer requires a different mindset—one focused on customers rather than providers. This shift can be difficult for many hospitals and health systems.

Conclusion

Succeeding with new payment models is not about demonstrating strong results in a short-term pilot demonstration project. It is about taking calculated risks and learning from successes and failures over the long term. It also requires making difficult decisions and having the courage to stay focused during challenging times. The organizations most likely to succeed recognize they are better off shaping their own future than waiting for it to happen. The benefits for providers and, most important, for the communities they serve will be well worth it.

References

Aon. 2015. "Third-Year Enrollment Results in the Aon Active Health Exchange Underscore Long-Term Sustainability of Private Exchanges." Press release. Issued May 6. http://ir.aon.com/about-aon/investor-relations/investor-news/news-release-details/2015/Third-Year-Enrollment-Results-in-the-Aon-Active-Health-Exchange-Underscore-Long-Term-Sustainability-of-Private-Exchanges/default.aspx.

Aon Hewitt. 2014. "Aon Hewitt Survey Shows US Employers Interested in Exploring Stricter Rules Around Health Benefits and Reference-Based Pricing as Part of Their Health Strategy." Press release. Issued June 11. http://aon.mediaroom.com/2014-06-11-Aon-Hewitt-Survey-Shows-U-S-Employers-Interested-in-Exploring-Stricter-Rules-Around-Health-Benefits-and-Reference-Based-Pricing-as-Part-of-their-Health-Strategy.

Birhanzel, R., S. Brown, and J. Tauber. 2015. "Private Health Insurance Exchange Enrollment Doubled from 2014 to 2015." Accessed September 14. www.accenture.com/us-en/insight-private-health-insurance-exchange-annual-enrollment.aspx.

Centers for Medicare & Medicaid Services (CMS). 2015. "Next Generation ACO Model." Updated November 2. https://innovation.cms.gov/initiatives/Next-Generation-ACO-Model/.

Herman, B. 2015. "More Health Systems Launch Insurance Plans Despite Caveats." *Modern Healthcare*. Published April 4. www.modernhealthcare.com/article/20150404/MAGAZINE/304049981.

Kaiser Family Foundation. 2014. "The Role of Medicare Advantage." Accessed September 24. http://kff.org/slideshow/the-role-of-medicare-advantage/.

US Department of Health & Human Services. 2015. "By the Numbers: Open Enrollment for Health Insurance." Published February 18. www.hhs.gov/healthcare/facts/factsheets/2015/02/open-enrollment-by-the-numbers.html.

There Is No Health(care) Without Mental Health(care)

by M. Justin Coffey, MD, and C. Edward Coffey, MD

A major opportunity to improve the value of healthcare in this country is to improve care for persons most vulnerable to receiving poor-quality care at high costs (Orszag and Emanuel 2010). The large and growing number of Americans who suffer from both mental and general medical disorders represents just such a population.

There Is No Health Without Mental Health

One in five Americans suffers from one or more mental disorders, most commonly anxiety, depression, and alcohol or substance abuse (Substance Abuse and Mental Health Services Administration 2012). Prevalence rates are nearly double among uninsured or Medicaid populations (Katon and Unützer 2013). The sheer pervasiveness of mental disorders contributes to high rates of comorbidity with general medical disorders. More than two-thirds of adults with a mental disorder have one or more chronic general medical disorders, and

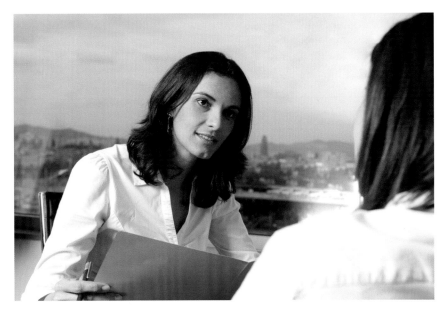

nearly one-third of adults with a chronic general medical disorder also suffer from a comorbid mental disorder (Alegria et al. 2003). In short, comorbidity is the rule rather than the exception.

Most mental disorders are chronic and potentially disabling, with four of

the top six causes for years lived with disability being some form of mental disorder (World Health Organization 2003). It comes as no surprise that a burden this severe brings with it deleterious effects on health outcomes. An extensive body of research has

About the Authors

M. Justin Coffey, MD, is a neuropsychiatrist who currently serves as medical director of the Center for Brain Stimulation at the Menninger Clinic in Houston, Texas, where he is also director of medical informatics. He is an associate professor of psychiatry and behavioral sciences at the Baylor College of Medicine. Dr. Coffey is a College Honors Scholar who attended the University of Chicago, where he earned a bachelor of arts degree in the history, philosophy, and social studies of science and medicine, as well as a medical degree. He completed a residency in psychiatry at the University of Michigan.

C. Edward Coffey, MD, is a neuropsychiatrist who currently serves as president and CEO of the Menninger Clinic in Houston, Texas. He is also a professor of psychiatry and behavioral sciences and of neurology at the Baylor College of Medicine. Dr. Coffey is a Rhodes Scholar who attended St. John's College, University of Oxford, England, where he earned a bachelor of arts degree focused on psychology, philosophy, and physiology after earning a bachelor of science degree in psychology from Wofford College in South Carolina. Dr. Coffey obtained his medical degree from Duke University, where he also completed residencies in neurology and psychiatry.

FUTURESCAN SURVEY RESULTS:
Behavioral Health

How likely is it that the following will be seen in your hospital's area by 2021?

Very Likely (%)	Somewhat Likely (%)	Somewhat Unlikely (%)	Very Unlikely (%)
26	41	24	10

More than 50 percent of primary care patients with a chronic general medical condition (e.g., diabetes, congestive heart failure, COPD) will receive some form of psychotherapy service (e.g., behavioral activation, motivational interviewing) that is embedded within primary care.

How likely is it that the following will be seen in **your hospital** by 2021?

Very Likely (%)	Somewhat Likely (%)	Somewhat Unlikely (%)	Very Unlikely (%)
9	42	35	14

More than 50 percent of your hospital's readmissions will be attributable to mental illness or psychosocial factors.

7	19	42	32

Admissions, transfers, or referrals to inpatient psychiatric care will be less than 50 percent of what they are today.

26	40	22	12

The proportion of your hospital's budget allocated to providing mental health care services will increase by 10 percentage points.

Note: Percentages may not total to exactly 100% due to rounding.

Behavioral Health: What Practitioners Predict

Primary care for chronic conditions will include psychotherapy services. About two-thirds (67 percent) of practitioners predict that within the next five years most patients in their hospital's area with a chronic illness will receive primary care that includes some type of psychotherapy service, such as behavioral activation or motivational interviewing.

Practitioners are divided about the role of mental illness and psychosocial issues among readmitted patients. Roughly half (51 percent) of practitioners surveyed think that by 2021 most of their hospital's readmissions will be attributable to mental illness or psychosocial factors, while about half (49 percent) hold an opposing view.

continued on pg. 45

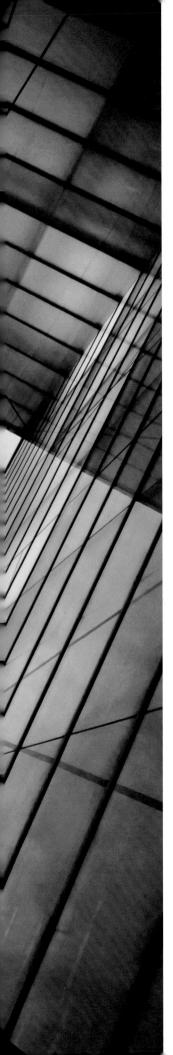

—continued from pg. 43

demonstrated that the comorbidity between mental disorders and general medical disorders increases symptom burden and functional impairment, impairs self-care (e.g., medication adherence, a healthy lifestyle), and decreases quality of life. What's worse, treatment for one disorder may exacerbate another. For example, medications used to treat bipolar disorder or schizophrenia can actually worsen diabetes by causing weight gain as well as problems with blood sugar and cholesterol metabolism. All in all, persons with comorbid mental and general medical disorders suffer a two- to fourfold increase in mortality, dying 25 years prematurely (Druss and Walker 2011).

There Is No Health*care* Without Mental Health*care*

Despite the prevalence of comorbid mental and general medical disorders, there are major gaps in the quality of care for affected patients. Mental disorders among persons with general medical disorders are underrecognized and undertreated, just as general medical disorders in persons with mental disorders are underrecognized and undertreated. Persons with comorbid mental and general medical disorders are less likely to receive preventive care, less likely to receive referrals to specialists when needed, and less likely to "land" at appointments with the specialists to whom they were referred (Katon and Unützer 2013).

These stark differences in quality of care exist despite the fact that this population accesses healthcare services frequently. Persons with comorbid mental and general medical disorders have higher rates of emergency department visits, as well as higher rates of rehospitalization for general medical disorders. In fact, they are recognized as "superutilizers" of healthcare services. A recent analysis of superutilizers in Denver County, Colorado, for example, found that more than 80 percent of patients identified as superutilizers were individuals with mental health disorders or multiple chronic disorders (Johnson et al. 2015).

These patterns of high utilization generate significantly higher costs of care. A person with depression and diabetes, for example, costs twice as much to care for as a person with diabetes alone, with the majority of the increase attributable to general medical expenditures (Simon et al. 2005). And because illnesses like depression are associated with disproportionate rates of absenteeism and productive days of work lost, employers share the burden of these increased costs (Goetzel et al. 2004).

With the passage of the Affordable Care Act, the need to deliver high-value, integrated care has become more urgent. The expansion of Medicaid will increase healthcare access for larger numbers of Americans with comorbid chronic mental and general medical disorders, and the passage of the Mental Health Parity and Addiction Equity Act will address limits on access to mental health care services. The era of accountability for population health has ushered in a new focus on designing delivery systems able to provide effective and efficient care for persons with comorbid mental and general medical disorders.

Integrating Mental Healthcare with General Medical Care Is Effective

Fortunately, models of integrated care exist, have been carefully and extensively studied, and have been shown to work for adults as well as for children and adolescents (Asarnow et al.

continued from pg. 44

Large reductions in inpatient psychiatric treatment are unlikely. Almost three-quarters (74 percent) of practitioners surveyed do not believe admissions, transfers, or referrals to inpatient psychiatric care will decrease by more than half by 2021.

Hospitals will allocate more of their budgets to providing mental health services. Almost two-thirds (66 percent) of survey respondents predict that the proportion of their budgets allocated to providing mental health services will increase by at least 10 percentage points over the next five years.

2015; Collins et al. 2010; Druss and Walker 2011). In primary care settings, integration tends to take place within the framework of the Chronic Care Model, a key aspect of which is effective clinical information systems (Butler et al. 2008). Such systems enable the active ingredients of integrated care, such as stepped care and the use of care managers, to have their positive effects (Bower et al. 2006; Katon et al. 2010). Outside of this framework, integration can take the form of colocation of services or facilitated referral. As reflected in the *Futurescan* survey results, the majority of healthcare leaders already predict that primary care will include traditional mental health care services, such as psychotherapy, particularly for patients with chronic disorders.

In the inpatient general medical setting, less is known about what types of models of integration can be effective. Generally, integration tends to involve embedding mental health clinicians (e.g., clinical social workers) in departments or services with a high volume of patients with mental illness (e.g., emergency departments). Less common are examples of integration between general hospitals and psychiatric hospitals, particularly when such hospitals serve the same patient population but are not part of the same healthcare system. The results from the *Futurescan* survey suggest that healthcare leaders recognize the need for integration at the hospital level. Just over half of survey respondents predict that more than 50 percent of rehospitalizations will be attributable to mental illness or psychosocial factors, and nearly 75 percent predict that the number of admissions, transfers, or referrals to psychiatric hospitals will increase.

Successful integration of mental and general medical healthcare can be cost-effective and help health systems achieve the Institute for Healthcare Improvement's Triple Aim of enhancing the patient experience, improving the health of populations, and reducing the cost of care (Archer et al. 2012). Nevertheless, adoption has been slow. Even among accountable care organizations, relatively little mental health care integration has occurred, with "contextual factors" cited as the main barrier (Lewis et al. 2014). Such contextual factors may only become more important, however, as the delivery of more and more mental health care services moves from hospitals and clinics to schools, prisons, nursing homes, and retail settings.

Implications for Healthcare Leaders

One key to successful mental health care integration is effective information management. Health system leaders can take important local steps now toward mental health care integration, even as they wait for payment models to evolve.

Establish a fully transparent medical record. For too long and in too many health systems, a "firewall" has prevented members of a patient's care team from accessing important and relevant mental health information about that patient. Shared information is a patient safety issue. For example, medications prescribed by a psychiatrist can affect a patient's general medical health. The Health Insurance Portability and Accountability Act (HIPAA) is often cited as a barrier to transparency, but HIPAA explicitly allows for the sharing of any and all clinical information that is pertinent to coordination of care. During the implementation of a new electronic health record (EHR) in the behavioral health services division of a large integrated healthcare system (the Henry Ford Health System), the team leading the project successfully eliminated firewalls that previously separated mental health care information from the rest of the patient's record, resulting in better communication among providers and dramatically higher quality of care for patients with mental health conditions (Coffey, Coffey, and Ahmedani 2013).

Design medical records in ways that facilitate the collection of behavioral and psychosocial information. Several behavioral factors (e.g., nicotine or alcohol use) and psychosocial factors (e.g., stress level, degree of social connectedness) are important determinants of health. Recognizing this important relationship, the Institute of Medicine (2014) has begun developing a framework for capturing social and behavioral information in EHRs. As health systems worldwide continue to implement electronic records, healthcare leaders would do well to ensure that such records efficiently gather and effectively display this information.

Pursue a pragmatic approach to screening for mental health conditions. Currently, little evidence supports universal screening for mental health disorders in primary care settings (O'Connor et al. 2009). An evidence-based approach to screening involves identifying those patients most at risk for having or developing a mental disorder and then screening only that subgroup of patients. In reality, however, designing, implementing, and following the processes necessary to identify which patients in a busy primary care clinic should be screened takes longer than simply screening every patient. A "non-evidence-based" approach may be more efficient, more easily adopted, and therefore more likely to be successful.

Conclusion

The results of the *Futurescan* survey indicate that two-thirds of healthcare leaders anticipate spending more in the next five years on mental health care delivery. One opportunity to maximize the return on that investment is to ensure that healthcare organizations have an information platform that facilitates the integration of mental and general medical healthcare.

References

Alegria, M., J.S. Jackson, R.C. Kessler, and D. Takeuchi. 2003. *National Comorbidity Survey Replication (NCS-R), 2001–2003*. Ann Arbor, MI: Inter-university Consortium for Political and Social Research.

Archer, J., P. Bower, S. Gilbody, K. Lovell, D. Richards, L. Gask, C. Dickens, and P. Coventry. 2012. "Collaborative Care for Depression and Anxiety Problems." *Cochrane Database of Systematic Reviews* 10: CD006525.

Asarnow, J.R., M. Rozenman, J. Wiblin, and L. Zeltzer. 2015. "Integrated Medical-Behavioral Care Compared with Usual Primary Care for Child and Adolescent Behavioral Health: A Meta-analysis." *JAMA Pediatrics* 169 (10): 929–37.

Bower, P., S. Gilbody, D. Richards, J. Fletcher, and A. Sutton. 2006. "Collaborative Care for Depression in Primary Care—Making Sense of a Complex Intervention: Systematic Review and Meta-regression." *British Journal of Psychiatry* 189 (6): 484–93.

Butler, M., R.L. Kane, D. McAlpine, R.G. Kathol, S.S. Fu, H. Hagedorn, and T.J. Wilt. 2008. *Integration of Mental Health/Substance Abuse and Primary Care*. AHRQ Publication No. 09-E003. Rockville, MD: Agency for Healthcare Research and Quality.

Coffey, C.E., M.J. Coffey, and B.K. Ahmedani. 2013. "An Update on Perfect Depression Care." *Psychiatric Services* 64 (4): 396.

Collins, C., D.L. Hewson, R. Munger, and T. Wade. 2010. *Evolving Models of Behavioral Health Integration in Primary Care*. New York: Millbank Memorial Fund.

Druss, B.G., and E.R. Walker. 2011. *Mental Disorders and Medical Comorbidity*. Princeton, NJ: Robert Wood Johnson Foundation.

Goetzel, R.Z., S.R. Long, R.J. Ozminkowski, K. Hawkins, S. Wang, and W. Lynch. 2004. "Health, Absence, Disability, and Presenteeism Cost Estimates of Certain Physical and Mental Health Conditions Affecting US Employers." *Journal of Occupational and Environmental Medicine* 46 (4): 398–412.

Institute of Medicine. 2014. *Capturing Social and Behavioral Domains in Electronic Health Records: Phase 1*. Washington, DC: National Academies Press.

Johnson, T.L., D.J. Rinehart, J. Durfee, D. Brewer, H. Batal, J. Blum, C.I. Oronce, and P. Melinkovich. 2015. "For Many Patients Who Use Large Amounts of Health Care Services, the Need Is Intense Yet Temporary." *Health Affairs* 34 (8): 1312–19.

Katon, W.J., E.H.B. Lin, M. Von Korff, P. Ciechanowski, E.J. Ludman, B. Young, D. Peterson, C. Rutter, M. McGregor, and D. McCulloch. 2010. "Collaborative Care for Patients with Depression and Chronic Illnesses." *New England Journal of Medicine* 363 (27): 2611–20.

Katon, W.J., and U. Unützer. 2013. "Health Reform and the Affordable Care Act: The Importance of Mental Health Treatment to Achieving the Triple Aim." *Journal of Psychosomatic Research* 74 (6): 533–37.

Lewis, V.A., C.H. Colla, K. Tierney, A.D. Van Critters, E.S. Fisher, and E. Meara. 2014. "Few ACOs Pursue Innovative Models That Integrate Care for Mental Illness and Substance Abuse with Primary Care." *Health Affairs* 33 (10): 1808–16.

O'Connor, E.A., E.P. Whitlock, B. Gaynes, and T.L. Beil. 2009. *Screening for Depression in Adults and Older Adults in Primary Care: An Updated Systematic Review*. AHRQ Publication No. 10-05143-EF-1. Rockville, MD: Agency for Healthcare Research and Quality.

Orszag, P.R., and E.J. Emanuel. 2010. "Health Care Reform and Cost Control." *New England Journal of Medicine* 363 (7): 601–2.

Simon, G.E., W.J. Katon, E.H. Lin, E. Ludman, M. Von Korff, P. Ciechanowski, and B.A. Young. 2005. "Diabetes complications and depression as predictors of health service costs." *General Hospital Psychiatry* 27 (5): 344–51.

Substance Abuse and Mental Health Services Administration. 2012. "State Estimates of Substance Use and Mental Disorders from the 2009–2010 National Surveys on Drug Use and Health." NSDUH Series H-43, HHS Publication No. (SMA) 12-4703. Rockville, MD: Substance Abuse and Mental Health Services Administration.

World Health Organization. 2003. "Investing in Mental Health." Geneva, Switzerland: World Health Organization.

Society for Healthcare Strategy & Market Development
Executive director: Diane Weber, RN
Senior editorial specialist: Brian Griffin

The Society for Healthcare Strategy & Market Development (SHSMD), a personal membership group of the American Hospital Association, is the largest and most prominent voice for healthcare professionals in strategic planning, marketing, public relations and communications. SHSMD is committed to helping its members prepare for the future with greater knowledge and opportunity as their organizations strive to improve the health and quality of life of their communities. The society serves more than 4,000 members by providing a broad and constantly updated array of resources, services, experiences and connections.

SHSMD leaders are available for on-site presentations about *Futurescan 2016–2021* to healthcare governing boards, senior management, planning teams and medical staffs. To arrange for a leadership presentation, contact the Society for Healthcare Strategy & Market Development at 312.422.3888 or shsmd@aha.org.

American College of Healthcare Executives/Health Administration Press
Executive vice president/COO: Elizabeth A. Summy, CAE
Director, Health Administration Press: Michael E. Cunningham
Survey: Leslie A. Athey and Peter Kimball
Project manager: Andrew J. Baumann
Layout editor: Cepheus Edmondson

The American College of Healthcare Executives is an international professional society of 40,000 healthcare executives who lead hospitals, healthcare systems and other healthcare organizations. ACHE's mission is to advance its members and healthcare management excellence. ACHE offers its prestigious FACHE® credential, signifying board certification in healthcare management. ACHE's established network of 80 chapters provides access to networking, education and career development at the local level. In addition, ACHE is known for its magazine, *Healthcare Executive*, and its career development and public policy programs. Through such efforts, ACHE works toward its vision of being the preeminent professional society for healthcare executives dedicated to improving health.

The Foundation of the American College of Healthcare Executives was established to further advance healthcare management excellence through education and research. The Foundation of ACHE is known for its educational programs—including the annual Congress on Healthcare Leadership, which draws more than 4,000 participants—and groundbreaking research. Its publishing division, Health Administration Press, is one of the largest publishers of books and journals on health services management, including textbooks for college and university courses. For more information, visit www.ache.org.

ABOUT THE SPONSOR
Evariant sees a future where healthcare organizations deliver efficient care solutions. We continuously innovate our healthcare CRM platform, based on a centralized communications engine capable of identifying, executing, and measuring all types of engagement initiatives. Results include greater visibility, richer engagement, and continuous improvement. Learn more at www.evariant.com. You can also follow Evariant on Twitter, Facebook and LinkedIn.